ELBOW ARTHROSCOPY

Elbow Arthroscopy

James R. Andrews, M.D.
Medical Director and Chairman
American Sports Medicine Institute
Orthopaedic Surgeon
Alabama Sports Medicine and Orthopaedic Center
Birmingham, Alabama

Stephen R. Soffer, M.D.
Team Physician
Albright College
Co-Director
Eastern Sports Medicine and Orthopedic Institute
Berkshire Orthopedic Associates, Inc.
Reading, Pennsylvania

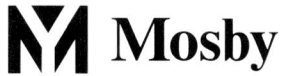

St. Louis Baltimore Boston Chicago London Madrid Philadelphia Sydney Toronto

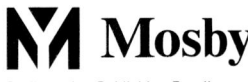
Mosby
Dedicated to Publishing Excellence

Publisher: *George Stamathis*
Editor: *Robert Hurley*
Associate Developmental Editor: *Lauranne Billus*
Assistant Director/Production, Editing, Design: *Frances Perveiler*
Project Manager: *Nancy C. Baker*
Proofroom Manager: *Barbara M. Kelly*
Designer: *Nancy C. Baker*
Manufacturing Supervisor: *Theresa Fuchs*

Copyright © 1994 by Mosby–Year Book, Inc.

All rights reserved. No part of this publication may be reproduced, stored in a retrieval system, or transmitted, in any form or by any means, electronic, mechanical, photocopying, recording, or otherwise, without prior written permission from the publisher.

Permission to photocopy or reproduce solely for internal or personal use is permitted for libraries or other users registered with the Copyright Clearance Center, provided that the base fee of $4.00 per chapter plus $.10 per page is paid directly to the Copyright Clearance Center, 27 Congress Street, Salem, MA 01970. This consent does not extend to other kinds of copying, such as copying for general distribution, for advertising or promotional purposes, for creating new collected works, or for resale.

Printed in the United States of America
Composition by Graphic World
Printing/binding by Walsworth

Mosby–Year Book, Inc.
11830 Westline Industrial Drive
St. Louis, Missouri 63146

Library of Congress Cataloging in Pubication Data

Andrews, James R. (James Reuben), 1942–
    Elbow arthroscopy / James R. Andrews, Stephen R. Soffer.
      p.   cm.
    Includes bibliographical references and index.
    ISBN 0-8016-7192-2
    1. Elbow—Endoscopic surgery. 2. Arthroscopy. I. Soffer,
Stephen R. II. Title.
    [DNLM: 1. Elbow Joint—surgery. 2. Arthroscopy—methods. WE 820
A567e 1993]
RD558.A53   1993
617.5'74—dc20
DNLM/DLC
for Library of Congress   93-30436
                                                                  CIP

1 2 3 4 5 6 7 8 9 0   98 97 96 95 94

We dedicate this text to both our teachers and students of elbow arthroscopy. Lanny Johnson has been an inspiration to us as well as all arthroscopists to pursue and explore new techniques in arthroscopic surgery. Jack Hughston has been a source of constant encouragement towards our endeavors to understand and expand on the knowledge of the shoulder and elbow. We would also like to thank our families for supporting us throughout our medical careers and specifically through this time-consuming process of publication.

Contributors

Richard L. Angelo, M.D.
Clinical Assistant Professor
Department of Orthopaedics
University of Washington
Evergreen General Medical Center
Kirkland, Washington

William G. Carson, Jr, M.D.
Clinical Assistant Professor of Orthopaedic Surgery
University of South Florida College of Medicine
Tampa, Florida

Scott D. Gillogly, M.D.
Clinical Assistant Professor of Surgery
Uniformed Services University of the Health Sciences
West Paces Medical Center
Atlanta, Georgia

Laura A. Timmerman, M.D.
Assistant Professor of Sports Medicine
Department of Orthopaedic Surgery
University of California, Davis, Medical Center
Sacramento, California

Kevin E. Wilk, P.T.
National Director of Research and Clinical Education
Healthsouth Rehabilitation Corporation
Associate Clinical Director
Healthsouth Sports Medicine and Rehabilitation Center
Director of Rehabilitation Research
American Sports Medicine Institute
Birmingham, Alabama

Preface

The elbow is a frequent site of pathology in sports injuries, work-related injuries, and degenerative disorders. However, our knowledge of the anatomy, biomechanics, and function of the elbow has only recently reached a stage of rapid expansion. As our understanding of the elbow increases, so does our desire and ability to treat these pathologies. Thus we have seen over the course of the last 10 years an increasing interest in elbow arthroscopy.

The goal of this endeavor was to develop a text that would aid those involved in the arthroscopic treatment of elbow injuries. The topics of anatomy, surgical indications, specific surgical arthroscopic techniques, complications, results, and postoperative rehabilitation are presented to allow the arthroscopist to perform elbow arthroscopy safely and effectively.

Elbow arthroscopic surgery and techniques are rapidly developing and changing. We hope this text serves as a means to consolidate present day information and also serve as a foundation for future advances.

We hope our readers find this text informative and helpful in the care of their patients and in the understanding of the principles of arthroscopic surgery of the elbow. We offer our best wishes to all those involved in the often challenging and rewarding endeavor of elbow arthroscopy.

Stephen R. Soffer, M.D.
James R. Andrews, M.D.

Acknowledgments

The process of publishing this text involved the efforts of many of our colleagues and friends. We would like to thank all of the chapter contributors for their fine work. We also would like to thank Linda Kimbrough for the beautiful color artwork as well as the line drawings. The efforts of the entire staff at American Sports Medicine Institute is also appreciated, and a special thanks to Dennis Dismukes, Jerry Conner, and Dale Baker.

Contents

Preface *xi*

1 / HISTORY OF ELBOW ARTHROSCOPY *1*
William G. Carson, Jr.

2 / INDICATIONS FOR ELBOW ARTHROSCOPY *5*
Scott D. Gillogly

3 / ELBOW ANATOMY RELATIVE TO ARTHROSCOPY *11*
Richard L. Angelo and Stephen R. Soffer

4 / DIAGNOSTIC ARTHROSCOPY OF THE ELBOW *33*
William G. Carson, Jr., Stephen R. Soffer, James R. Andrews

5 / ARTHROSCOPIC SURGICAL PROCEDURES OF THE ELBOW: COMMON CASES *59*
Stephen R. Soffer and James R. Andrews

6 / ARTHROSCOPIC SURGICAL PROCEDURES OF THE ELBOW: UNCOMMON CASES *87*
Stephen R. Soffer and James R. Andrews

7 / COMPLICATIONS OF ELBOW ARTHROSCOPY *101*
William G. Carson, Jr.

8 / REHABILITATION OF THE ELBOW IN THROWING ATHLETES *109*
Kevin E. Wilk

9 / CLINICAL EXPERIENCE *131*
Laura A. Timmerman and James R. Andrews

Index *141*

Chapter 1

History of Elbow Arthroscopy

William G. Carson, Jr., M.D.

Arthroscopy of the elbow is a useful and effective procedure that has its foundation in the popular techniques of knee and shoulder arthroscopy. Because of technical advances in arthroscopic equipment, the development of various arthroscopic techniques for elbow arthroscopy,[2, 3, 5, 8, 15, 20] and the existing knowledge of arthroscopic anatomy of the elbow, the procedure is now well-established. The value of diagnostic elbow arthroscopy is widely accepted, and the visualization obtained with arthroscopy far exceeds that obtained even with multiple arthrotomies about this joint.

Arthroscopy of the elbow is a technically demanding surgical procedure, and attention to detail is essential for a safe and reproducible arthroscopic examination. A thorough knowledge of the extraarticular portal anatomy of the elbow is necessary because the arthroscopic instruments must be placed through deep muscle layers and near important neurovascular structures. Injury to nearby neurovascular structures about the elbow is possible, and other anatomic barriers exist, such as a tightly constrained joint that precludes marked distention or manipulation to improve visualization or advancement of arthroscopic instruments.

Because of the technical intricacies of elbow arthroscopy and the proximity of neurovascular structures in performance of elbow arthroscopy, the majority of orthopedic surgeons who perform arthroscopic surgery do not perform elbow arthroscopy. In a study conducted by the American Academy of Orthopaedic Surgeons (Fig 1–1), it was found that approximately 81% of orthopedic surgeons in the United States perform some type of arthroscopic surgery. It was estimated that 77% performed arthroscopic procedures in the knee, 42% in the shoulder, 25% in the ankle, 12% in the elbow, and 8% in the wrist. This same survey found that 81% of the actual surgical procedures were performed in the knee, 12% in the shoulder, 4% in the ankle, 2% in the elbow, and 2% in the wrist.

EVOLUTION OF ELBOW ARTHROSCOPY

The first mention of arthroscopy of the elbow in the orthopedic literature was by Michael Burman[4] in 1931. At that time he reported on arthroscopy performed with a 3-mm-diameter endoscope in cadavers. He stated that the elbow was "unsuitable for examination" and that "anterior puncture of the elbow is out of the question." In 1971, Watanabe[23] developed the 1.7-mm no. 24 arthroscope for use in small joints. After this development, various surgical approaches to elbow arthroscopy were described, including those of Ito[12, 13] and Maeda,[17] in 1979 and 1980. In 1981, Ito[14] reported a clinical study

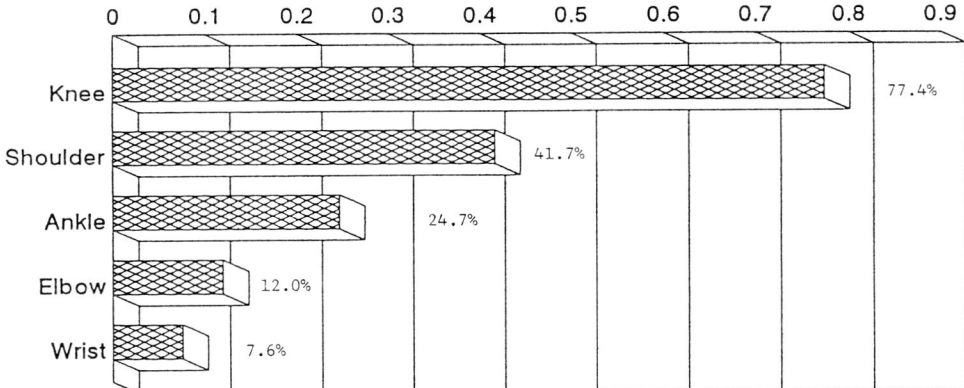

FIG 1-1. Percentage of orthopedic surgeons performing arthroscopic procedures by anatomic site. Overall, 81.2% of orthopedic surgeons indicated they performed arthroscopic procedures. Fewer than 1% performed arthroscopy of the hip or spine. (Data from 1990 Orthopaedic Physician Census, Supplemental Form B, American Academy of Orthopaedic Surgeons.)

(226 cases) of elbow arthroscopy in the Japanese literature. In 1983 in the European literature, Hempfling[11] described the prone position for elbow arthroscopy; and in 1989, Poehling et al.[20] described the prone approach combined with a proximal medial arthroscopic portal. In 1985, Guhl[10] reported on a series of 45 elbow arthroscopies. Also in 1985, Andrews and Carson[1] reported on 12 cases of elbow arthroscopy and reviewed the arthroscopic technique and anatomy of the elbow. Johnson[15] has presented excellent descriptions of the technique of elbow arthroscopy and intraarticular pathologic conditions.

In addition to the multiple reports concerning arthroscopy of the elbow, various instructional courses have been presented, including those by the American Academy of Orthopaedic Surgeons,[7, 18] the Arthroscopy Association of North America, and the American Orthopaedic Society for Sports Medicine.

As elbow arthroscopy became more common and the indications were expanded, the incidence of neurovascular complications appeared to increase. In 1986, Lynch et al.[16] performed cadaver studies demonstrating the extraarticular portal anatomy and the proximity of neurovascular structures. Also in 1986, Small[21] reviewed the complications of arthroscopic surgery, including arthroscopy performed in small joints such as the elbow. Casscells[9] and Thomas et al.[22] reviewed complications of elbow arthroscopy in 1987, and Carson[6] and Papilion et al.[19] reviewed various arthroscopic complications and performed literature reviews in 1988.

SUMMARY

Diagnostic and surgical arthroscopy of the elbow have now been well established, and the interest in this surgical procedure continues to increase. The future of elbow arthroscopy depends on its continued effectiveness in diagnosis and treatment of certain disorders in and around the elbow, such as osteochondritis dissecans of the capitellum or loose bodies around the elbow. Its future also depends on an acceptably low complication rate, particularly regarding neurovascular complications.

REFERENCES

1. Andrews JR, Carson WG: Arthroscopy of the elbow, *Arthroscopy*, 1:97–107, 1985.
2. Andrews JR, Carson WG: Arthroscopy of the elbow. In McGinty JB, editor: *Techniques in orthopaedics: arthroscopic surgery update.* Rockville, Md, 1985, Aspen Systems, pp 183–190.
3. Andrews JR, St. Pierre RK, Carson WG: Arthroscopy of the elbow, *Clin Sports Med* 5:653–662, 1986.
4. Burman MS: Arthroscopy or the direct visualization of joints, *J Bone Joint Surg* 13:669–695, 1931.
5. Carson WG, Andrews JR: Arthroscopy of the elbow. In Zarins B, Andrews JR, Carson WG, editors: *Injuries to the throwing arm*, Philadelphia, 1985, WB Saunders, pp 221–227.
6. Carson WG: Complications of elbow arthroscopy. In Minkoff J, Sherman O, editors: *Arthroscopic surgery*, Baltimore, 1988, Williams & Wilkins.
7. Carson WG: Arthroscopy of the elbow, *Instr Course Lect* 37:195–201, 1988.
8. Carson WG, Meyers JF: Diagnostic arthroscopy of the elbow: surgical technique and arthroscopic and portal anatomy. In McGinty JB, editor: *Operative arthroscopy*, New York, 1991, Raven Press, pp 583–594.
9. Casscells SW: Neurovascular anatomy and elbow arthroscopy: inherent risks, editor's comment, *Arthroscopy* 2:190, 1987.
10. Guhl JF: Arthroscopy and arthroscopic surgery of the elbow, *Orthopedics* 8:290–296, 1985.
11. Hempfling H: Die endoskopische Untersuching des Ellenbogengelenkes vom dorsoradialen Zugang. *Z Orthop* 121:331, 1983.
12. Ito K: The arthroscopic anatomy of the elbow joint, *Arthroscopy* 4:2–9, 1979 (Japanese literature).
13. Ito K: Arthroscopy of the elbow joint: a cadaver study, *Arthroscopy* 5:9–22, 1980. (Japanese literature)
14. Ito K: Arthroscopy of the elbow joint, *Arthroscopy* 6:15–24, 1981.
15. Johnson LL: Elbow arthroscopy. In *Arthroscopic surgery: principles and practice*, St Louis, 1986, Mosby, pp 1446–1477.
16. Lynch GJ, Meyers JF, Whipple TL, et al: Neurovascular anatomy and elbow arthroscopy; inherent risks, *Arthroscopy* 2:191–197, 1986.
17. Maeda Y: Arthroscopy of the elbow joint, *Arthroscopy* 5:5–8, 1980. (Japanese literature)
18. Morrey BF: Arthroscopy of the elbow, *Instr Course Lect* 35:102, 1986.
19. Papilion JD, Neff RS, Shall LM: Compression neuropathy of the radial nerves as a complication of elbow arthroscopy: a case report and review of the literature, *Arthroscopy* 4:284–286, 1988.
20. Poehling GG, Whipple TL, Sisco L, et al: Elbow arthroscopy: a new technique, *Arthroscopy* 5:222–224, 1989.
21. Small NC: Complication in arthroscopy: on knee and other joints, *Arthroscopy* 2:253–258, 1986.
22. Thomas MA, Fast A, Shapiro D: Radial nerve damage as a complication to elbow arthroscopy, *Clin Orthop* 215:130–131, 1987.
23. Watanabe M: Arthroscopy of small joints, *J Jpn Orthop Assoc* 45:908, 1979. (Japanese literature)

Chapter 2

Indications for Elbow Arthroscopy

Scott D. Gillogly, M.D.

Significant experience with elbow arthroscopy has been limited to the past decade. However, as experience with elbow arthroscopy grew, the indications for its use gradually expanded. Technologic advances in arthroscopic equipment and surgical techniques have permitted orthopedists to perform more intricate procedures arthroscopically. From 1986 through 1992, more than 25 articles have been published on various aspects of elbow arthroscopy, further defining and expanding its indications. Safety has been enhanced through further anatomic studies and alternate operative techniques.[13, 15, 21] In this chapter, we discuss the current indications for elbow arthroscopy, as well as the contraindications, including:

1. Loose bodies.
2. Osteochondritis dissecans
3. Chronic synovitis (e.g., repetitive trauma, rheumatoid arthritis, synovial osteochondromatosis, lateral synovial plica)
4. Osteoarthritis, posttraumatic arthritis
5. Valgus extension overload syndrome
6. Acute injury and fracture
7. Adhesions and contractures
8. Septic arthritis
9. Undiagnosed painful elbow (e.g., evaluation of ulnar collateral ligament, new onset flexion contracture, elbow snapping, biopsy)

LOOSE BODIES

Extraction of loose bodies from the elbow was the first notable indication for operative elbow arthroscopy.* This less invasive technique offered much less operative morbidity than the more conventional arthrotomy. The excellent early clinical success of operative elbow arthroscopy in removal of loose bodies paved the way for further indications.

Loose bodies may be either chondral and found incidentally within the elbow joint during arthroscopy or osteochondral and appear on plain radiographs or computed tomography scans. Patients may have intermittent motion deficits, locking, or clicking symptoms. Loose bodies may rest in the anterior, lateral, or posterior compartments,

*References 1, 2, 4, 7, 8, 10, 12, 14, 16, 17, 28.

although they tend to be in the compartment of the causative pathologic feature. Therefore, loose bodies are more likely to be posterior in a throwing athlete with chronic valgus extension overload syndrome (VEOS), and anterior or lateral in a patient with Panner's disease.[3, 22] Loose bodies may be attached to the synovium or move freely around the joint. Chondral or osteochondral loose bodies are easily amenable to treatment by arthroscopic removal, thus avoiding the use of arthrotomy.*

OSTEONCHONDRITIS DISSECANS AND PANNER'S DISEASE

Panner's disease is an idiopathic disorder of the endochondral ossification of the capitellar epiphysis. This osteochondrosis usually occurs in preadolescent boys, and may or may not be associated with some form of trauma.[22] Osteochondritis dissecans usually occurs in an adolescent patient involved in an activity placing high shear and compressive loads across the radiocapitellar joint, such as baseball throwing or gymnastics.[11, 20, 22] The distinction between these two processes may be artificial, because they may represent different presentations of the same underlying idiopathic osteochondrosis.

Patients with either of these processes may have joint incongruities caused by chondral or osteochondral defects, loose bodies, and reactive synovitis. Lesions predominantly involve the capitellum, but may secondarily affect the radial head.[1, 2, 11, 20, 22] When lesions are unresponsive to nonoperative treatment, elbow arthroscopy allows removal of joint debris and loose bodies and debridement of hypertrophic synovium.† Also, curettage or drilling of osteochondral defects and possibly pinning or some other form of fixation of replaceable, large osteochondral fragments can be performed arthroscopically.‡

CHRONIC SYNOVITIS

Patients with repetitive trauma, rheumatoid arthritis, synovial osteochondromatosis, lateral synovial plica, and inflammatory arthritides all will have elbow pain resulting from reactive synovitis either as a primary or secondary process. The beneficial effects of synovectomy in inflammatory arthritis have been demonstrated in other joints and are equally applicable in the elbow. Arthroscopy provides the common avenue to treat these diverse pathologic processes.

In rheumatoid arthritis, considerable pain relief can be achieved through a near complete synovectomy, provided that articular cartilage and the underlying bone have not been extensively destroyed by the rheumatoid process.[2, 5, 8, 24, 28] The effects may be transient, but the less invasive arthroscopic technique may be a much more attractive alternative than open synovectomy.

The primary synovial process of synovial chondromatosis can also be addressed arthroscopically, allowing removal of the multiple cartilaginous loose bodies as well as nearly complete synovectomy.[19, 28] Debridement of the metaplastic synovium is the primary treatment of this disorder, although recurrences are relatively common (see Chapter 6). Another primary process of the synovium that is amenable to arthroscopic treatment in the elbow is pigmented villonodular synovitis.

A lateral synovial plica has been noted in the elbow near the radial head and capitellar articulation. This synovial fringe or fold may represent a septal remnant, which has been

---

*References 2, 4, 7, 8, 9, 12, 14, 16, 17, 28.
†References 2, 8, 11, 12, 17, 18, 19, 22, 28.
‡References 2, 8, 11, 12, 22, 28.

described in the knee, and has been implicated as a source of symptoms in tennis elbow. Its open excision has been described.[6] Several cases implicating this lateral synovial fringe or plica as a cause of elbow pain mimicking a loose body have been reported, with good clinical response to arthroscopic excision of the fibrotic lateral synovial plica.[6, 24]

Patients with chronic synovitis secondary to repetitive trauma or overuse, when unresponsive to conservative treatment, may experience relief of symptoms with limited arthroscopic debridement of hypertrophic synovium. These patients may also benefit from arthroscopic intervention, on the basis of undiagnosed painful elbow.[2, 5, 8, 19, 28] The extent of elbow synovitis cannot be adequately assessed before such an operation. In addition to the benefit of visual inspection afforded by arthroscopy, the procedure also provides the opportunity for performance of synovial biopsy, to aid in establishment of the correct diagnosis.[19] This is especially helpful in inflammatory arthritides, such as rheumatoid arthritis, ankylosing spondylitis, pseudogout, Reiter's syndrome, psoriatic arthritis, and monoarticular seronegative rheumatoid arthritis.[2, 19]

OSTEOARTHRITIS AND POSTTRAUMATIC ARTHRITIS

The effects of arthroscopic lavage, removal of debris, and debridement of chondral fibrillations and fragmentation in patients with degenerative or posttraumatic arthritis of the elbow provide relief similar to that in other joints.* The lasting beneficial effects, however, need further investigation. An increase in motion gained by excising osteophytes and spurs in these conditions has been beneficial at short-term follow-up. When the symptoms stem predominantly from loose bodies, debris, and loss of motion secondary to osteoarthritic spurring, removal and lavage provide good relief.[2, 19, 24] Disease in patients with degenerative arthritis tends to be more diffuse than the more isolated reactive joint changes that might occur in the posterior compartment in VEOS or the anterior compartment in osteochondritis dissecans.

Abrasion chondroplasty for chondromalacia of the radial head or capitellum has shown marginal results, both objectively and subjectively.[2] Diagnosis of the degree and location of involvement and lavage of loose debris may have the most beneficial effects on chondromalacia and early degenerative joint diseases.[2, 5, 19, 24] Activity modification, administration of nonsteroidal antiinflammatory drugs (NSAIDS), and rehabilitation emphasizing stretching, strengthening, and obtaining full range of motion and flexibility remain the treatment alternatives.

VALGUS EXTENSION OVERLOAD SYNDROME

The rapid and forceful elbow extension generated during throwing generates high compressive loads on the posterior olecranon articulation. This load is particularly concentrated on the posterior medial portion of the olecranon because of the valgus moment about the elbow during the acceleration phase of throwing. These repetitive stresses produce osteochondral changes and hypertrophy of the olecranon process, as well as of the trochlear articulation, with eventual articular incongruity and loss of terminal extension.[1, 3]

When a throwing athlete diagnosed as having VEOS fails to respond to several months of conservative treatment of rest, NSAID therapy, and a supervised rehabilitation program,

*References 2, 5, 8, 19, 24, 28.

elbow arthroscopy is the next treatment of choice. During routine assessment of the anterior compartment as well, loose bodies, hypertrophic synovium, osteochondral defects, and osteophytes can frequently be demonstrated in the posterior compartment. This condition responds to debris and loose body removal, and debridement lesions with osteotomes and arthroscopic shavers and burrs.[2, 3, 5] Careful attention needs to be directed to the close proximity of the ulnar nerve.[2, 5] Recurrence of this syndrome, even after successful initial treatment, is not unusual.[2, 3]

ACUTE INJURY AND FRACTURE

The usefulness of arthroscopy in acute elbow trauma appears to be less distinct than other indications, but several potential situations exist.[2, 5, 8, 19, 28] First, the degree of displacement or articular stepoff can be assessed in equivocal cases, to establish the need for further open reduction and internal fixation vs. excision of the fractured radial head. Treatment decisions regarding subtle fractures of the radial head and capitellum may benefit from arthroscopic assessment. In acute fractures, however, intraosseous bleeding into the joint can obscure visualization and make the procedure nondiagnostic.[19] Arthroscopic removal of chondral or osteochondral fragments may restore motion when acute fracture produces fragments that block motion. Although arthroscopic fixation of acute fractures with percutaneous pins has been described, it appears to be useful in only a select type of fracture.[2, 12, 19, 28] The literature and our personal experience with arthroscopic reduction and internal fixation are quite limited. Further investigation is necessary before clear indications can be recommended.

ADHESIONS AND CONTRACTURES

Loss of motion in the elbow can be the result of bone or soft tissue problems. The motion loss is a reflection of the underlying pathologic process, which may be focal or diffuse within the elbow. Resection of bony osteophytes in degenerative processes in an attempt to gain motion has shown only modest success.[2, 5, 8, 24, 28] Debridement of intraarticular adhesions after a hemarthrosis, acute injury, or other inflammatory process seems to produce better improvements in motion.[2, 5, 19, 24] Arthroscopic lysis of adhesions gives better gains with flexion than with extension or pronation and supination.[2, 24] Successful results have been reported after arthroscopic debridement of adhesions associated with motion deficits and snapping after excision of the radial head.[2, 19]

SEPTIC ARTHRITIS

The advantages of arthroscopic treatment in an early stage of sepsis have been well documented in the knee. These advantages include lower surgical morbidity, minimal scarring, and earlier return to functional activities. Arthroscopic debridement of adhesions and necrotic tissue, copious lavage and joint distention, and placement of drainage tubes are factors important to improved results in treatment of knee sepsis. The advantages in the knee certainly could be reproduced in the septic elbow. Although no series of arthroscopic treatment of the septic elbow have been reported, several cases (as well as ruled out cases) have been reported as parts of series of elbow arthroscopies.[19, 23, 24]

UNDIAGNOSED PAINFUL ELBOW

In patients with chronic elbow pain and no demonstrable lesion on radiographic or other imaging studies, arthroscopy can be useful in establishing or ruling out treatable diagnoses. Some authors have suggested that identification of some lesions, especially chondral surface defects and degenerative arthroses, may be the most important aspect of management, because it allows appropriate patient counseling and avoidance of aggravating activities.[2, 5] This is most advantageous in lesions such as advanced chondromalacia, where further intervention with chondroplasty provides little long-term benefit.[2, 5] Conversely, in patients with no demonstrable intraarticular lesion, the benefit may be recommendations for more rapid rehabilitation and return to normal activity.[2, 5, 19]

Painful conditions that can be delineated with diagnostic arthroscopy include unrecognized cartilaginous loose bodies, osteochondritis dissecans, posttraumatic arthritis, adhesions, subtle VEOS, and joint surface incongruity. In conditions including inflammatory synovitis, synovial biopsy may provide the elusive diagnosis.[19]

Another often difficult diagnostic entity is ulnar collateral ligament tear or laxity. The ulnar collateral ligament arthroscopic stress test[26] will show widening between the ulna and distal humerus during anterior compartment arthroscopy (see Chapter 5). Also, the posterior band may be visualized arthroscopically from the posterior compartment.

A recent study from the Mayo Clinic has demonstrated a useful diagnostic yield of 64% among 56 planned elbow arthroscopies.[19] Overall, the researchers believed that 51 of 70 patients (73%) who underwent arthroscopy benefited in some way. The yield was much lower in patients who had normal results at radiography and physical examination, and the clinical management was not affected.[19] Arthroscopy was particularly recommended in cases of spontaneous flexion contracture and elbow snapping. The cause of snapping was identified with diagnostic arthroscopy in 11 of 12 patients, and further arthroscopic treatment was successful in six of those.[19]

CONTRAINDICATIONS TO ELBOW ARTHROSCOPY

Despite initial concerns regarding the safety of elbow arthroscopy, surprisingly few major complications have been reported.[5, 13, 15, 19, 24, 25, 27] This, along with the proved efficacy of arthroscopy in many diverse conditions involving the elbow, has gradually expanded the clinical indications, while relative contraindications have diminished.

Contraindications include conditions in which the normal bone architecture and soft tissue anatomy have been distorted to the extent that the neurovascular structures cannot reliably be avoided or the intraarticular space precludes visualization and instrumentation. Such conditions affecting the joint architecture may include bony ankylosis or severe fibrous ankylosis. Previous surgery such as nerve transposition or osteotomy may alter the normal portal anatomy and place neurovascular structures at risk.[5]

SUMMARY

Although arthroscopy of the elbow is technically demanding, it seems to offer many advantages across a wide spectrum of elbow conditions, with minimal risk. As experience broadens, indications no doubt will expand. As more clinical follow-up is reported, the indications will be better refined and more accurate prognostic data will be available to the surgeon.

REFERENCES

1. Andrews JR: Bony injuries about the elbow in the throwing athlete, *Instr Course Lect* 34:323–331, 1985.
2. Andrews JR, Carson WG: Arthroscopy of the elbow, *Arthroscopy* 1:97–107, 1985.
3. Andrews JR, Craven WM: Lesions of the posterior compartment of the elbow, *Clin Sports Med* 10:637–652, 1991.
4. Boe S: Arthroscopy of the elbow: diagnosis and extraction of loose bodies, *Acta Orthop Scand* 57:52–53, 1986.
5. Carson WG: Arthroscopy of the elbow, *Instr Course Lect* 37:195–201, 1988.
6. Clarke RP: Symptomatic, lateral synovial fringe (plica) of the elbow joint, *Arthroscopy* 4:112–116, 1988.
7. Faulkner JR, Jackson RW: Arthroscopy of the elbow, *J Bone Joint Surg [Br]* 62:130, 1980.
8. Guhl JF: Arthroscopy and arthroscopic surgery of the elbow, *Orthopedics* 8:1290–1296, 1985.
9. Hempfling H: Endoscopic examination of the elbow joint from the dorsoradial approach, *Z Orthop* 121:331–332, 1983.
10. Hempfling H: Arthroscopy of the elbow joint: indications and results, *Z Orthop* 122:750–753, 1984.
11. Jackson DW, Silvino N, Reiman P: Osteochondritis in the female gymnast's elbow, *Arthroscopy* 5:129–136, 1989.
12. Johnson LL: *Diagnostic and surgical arthroscopy: the knee and other joints,* ed 2, St Louis, 1981, Mosby.
13. Lindenfeld TN: Medial approach in elbow arthroscopy, *Am J Sports Med* 18:413–417, 1990.
14. Lokietek JC, De Cloedt, F Legaye J, et al: Extraction of a foreign body from the elbow using arthroscopy, *Rev Chir Orthop* 74:93–98, 1988.
15. Lynch GJ, Meyers JF, Whipple TL, et al: Neurovascular anatomy and elbow arthroscopy; inherent risks, *Arthroscopy* 2:190–197, 1986.
16. McGinty JB: Arthroscopic removal of loose bodies, *Orthop Clin North Am* 13:313–328, 1982.
17. Morrey BF: Arthroscopy of the elbow. In Morrey BF, editor: *The elbow and its disorders,* Philadelphia, 1985, WB Saunders, pp 115–121.
18. Morrey BF: Arthroscopy of the elbow, *Instr Course Lect* 35:102–107, 1986.
19. O'Driscoll SW, Morrey BF: Arthroscopy of the elbow: diagnostic and therapeutic benefits and hazards, *J Bone Joint Surg [Am]* 74:84–94, 1992.
20. Pappas AM: Osteochondrosis dissecans. *Clin Orthop* 158:59–69, 1981.
21. Poehling GG, Whipple TL, Sisco L, et al: Elbow arthroscopy: a new technique, *Arthroscopy* 5:222–224, 1989.
22. Ruch DS, Poehling GG: Arthroscopic treatment of Panner's disease, *Clin Sports Med* 10:629–636, 1991.
23. Shaffer B, Parisien JS: Elbow arthroscopy, *Surg Rounds Orthop* 3:113–117, 1989.
24. Sheppard JE, Marion JD, Hurst DI: Arthroscopic elbow surgery: five year experience and observations in 48 cases, *Am J Arthroscopy* 1:13–19, 1991.
25. Small N: Complications in arthroscopy: the knee and other joints, *Arthroscopy* 2:253–258, 1986.
26. Soffer SR, Andrews JR: The ulnar collateral ligament arthroscopic stress test. Presented at American Academy of Orthopaedic Surgeons 61st annual meeting, March 1994, New Orleans.
27. Thomas MA, Fast A, Shapiro D: Radial nerve damage as a complication of elbow arthroscopy, *Clin Orthop* 215:130–131, 1987.
28. Woods GW: Elbow arthroscopy, *Clin Sports Med* 6:557–564, 1987.

Chapter 3

Elbow Anatomy Relative to Arthroscopy

Richard L. Angelo, M.D.
Stephen R. Soffer, M.D.

After studying cadaver elbows with a 3.0-mm endoscope in 1931, Burman[2] concluded that the elbow was "unsuitable for examination" and that "anterior puncture of the elbow is out of the question." Through careful study of the anatomy in and around the elbow, Ito,[5,6] Maeda,[10] and others[1,4,7] have since demonstrated that arthroscopy of the elbow can be successfully and safely performed. Elbow arthroscopy is a precise and demanding technique, and because of the proximity of important neurovascular structures to the recommended portals, the surgeon must be thoroughly familiar with elbow anatomy. Also, the high degree of congruency of the articular surfaces and the relatively small capsular volume make sound arthroscopic skills a necessity. This chapter describes the features of elbow anatomy that are of significance to surgeons performing elbow arthroscopy.

GROSS ANATOMY

An appreciation of the superficial anatomy of the elbow enables the surgeon to accurately identify important landmarks to serve as guides in safe establishment of arthroscopic portals. Three muscular borders on the anterior aspect of the elbow outline the antecubital fossa (Fig 3–1). The lateral margin is formed by the wrist extensors, or "mobile wad" of Henry, and includes the brachioradialis, extensor carpi radialis longus, and extensor carpi radialis brevis, which originate from the lateral epicondyle. The extensor digitorum communis, extensor digiti minimi, and extensor carpi ulnaris originate from the lateral epicondyle further posterolaterally (Fig 3–2). The medial border of the cubital fossa is formed by the pronator teres, which originates from the medial epicondyle along with the flexor carpi radialis, flexor digitorum superficialis, palmaris longus, and flexor carpi ulnaris. The superior extent of the fossa is defined by the biceps muscle. Its lacertus fibrosis creates a roof, and the brachialis and supinator muscles form the floor of the fossa.

The lateral epicondyle and more prominent medial epicondyle of the humerus, as well as the olecranon process of the proximal ulna, are readily palpable (Fig 3–3). From a posterior view, these three landmarks nearly form a transverse line when the elbow is

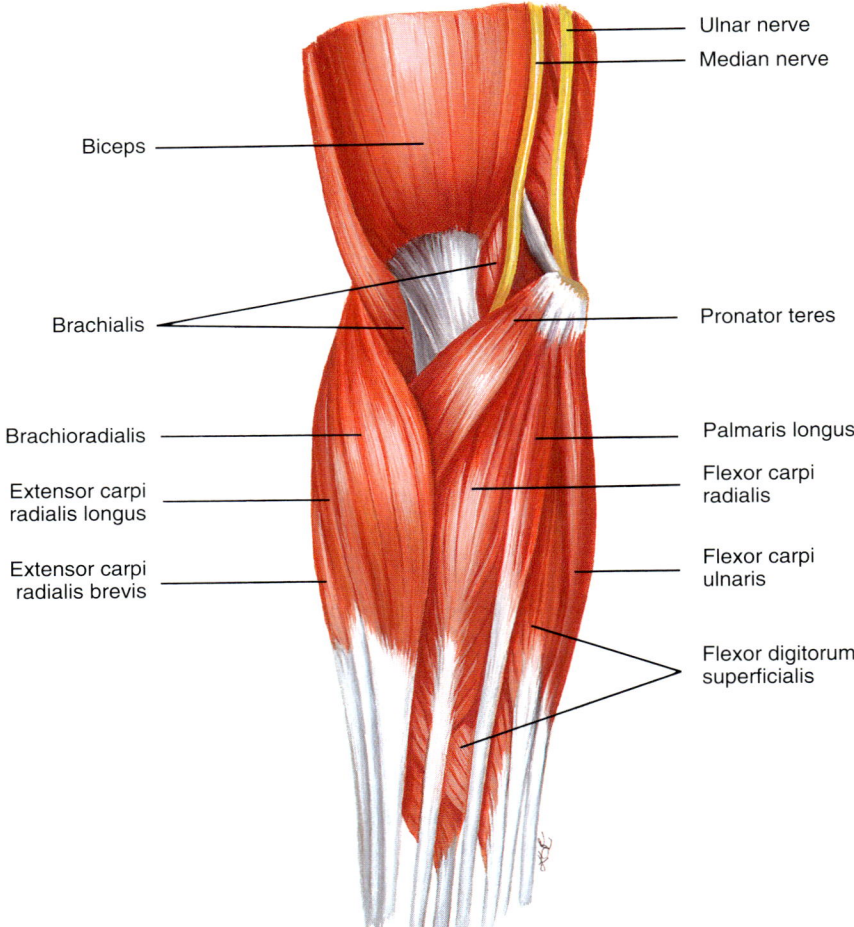

FIG 3–1. Anterior aspect of right elbow (antecubital fossa).

in extension, and form an inverted equilateral triangle when the elbow is flexed to 90 degrees[11] (Fig 3–4). Anteriorly, a line joining the epicondyles runs approximately at the level of the flexion crease. One centimeter distal to this line in the anterior midline lies the imaginary center of the elbow joint (Fig 3–5). By pronating and supinating the forearm, the radial head may be easily palpated several centimeters distal to the lateral epicondyle. On the lateral aspect of the elbow a second equilateral triangle is formed by the lateral epicondyle, olecranon, and radial head (Fig 3–6). At the center of this triangle is the "soft spot," through which aspiration and distention of the elbow with fluid are performed in preparation for arthroscopy.

The posterior surface of the elbow is composed proximally of the triceps muscle and its broad tendinous insertion (see Fig 3–2). Posterolaterally, the anconeus muscle originates on the lateral epicondyle and posterior elbow capsule and inserts on the proximal ulna.

Just medial to the biceps tendon in the middle of the antecubital fossa, the brachial arterial pulse may be palpated. The cephalic and basilic veins course over the anterior aspect of the elbow and are the most prominent veins of the variable superficial venous complex.

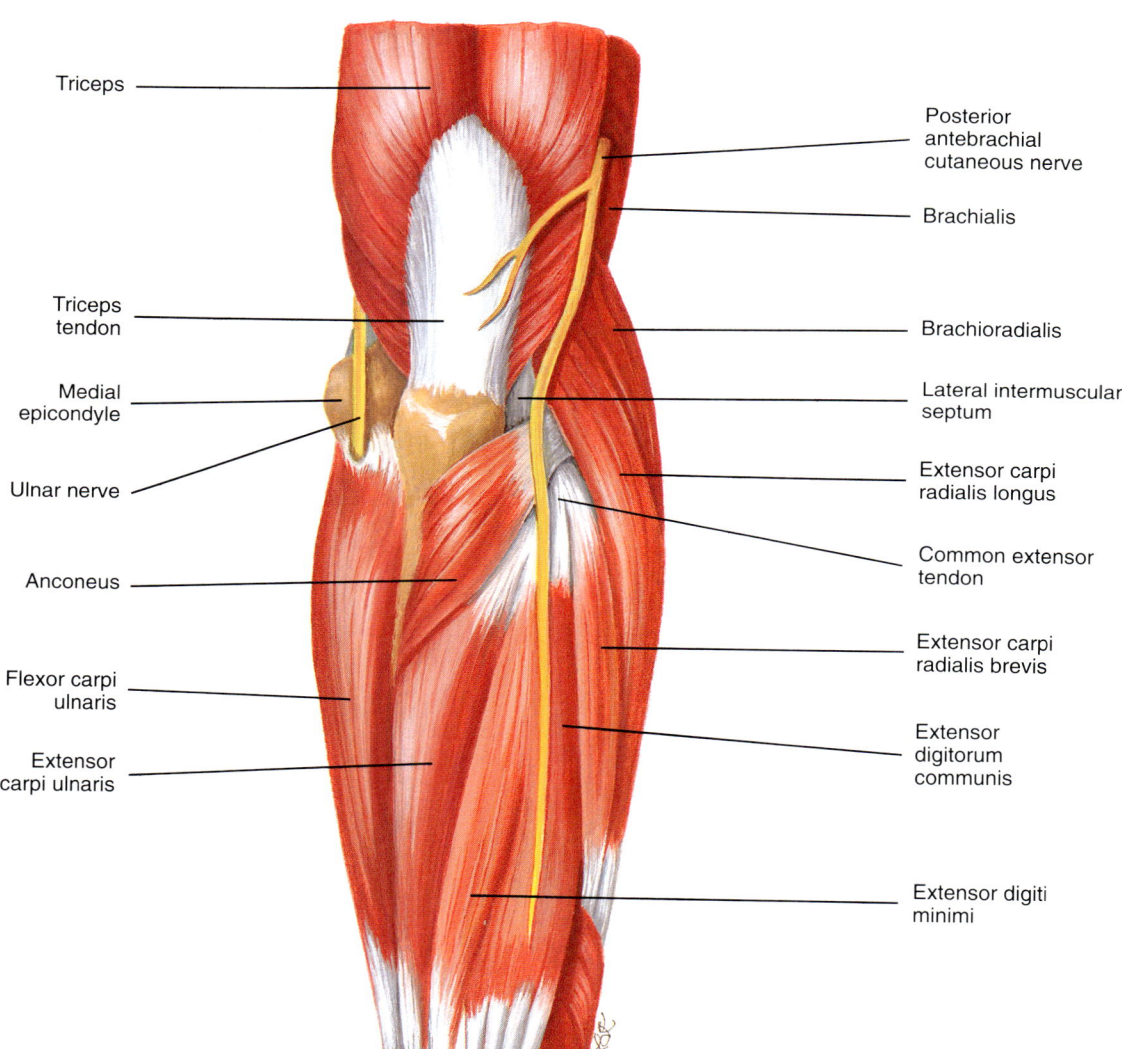

FIG 3–2. Posterior aspect of the elbow.

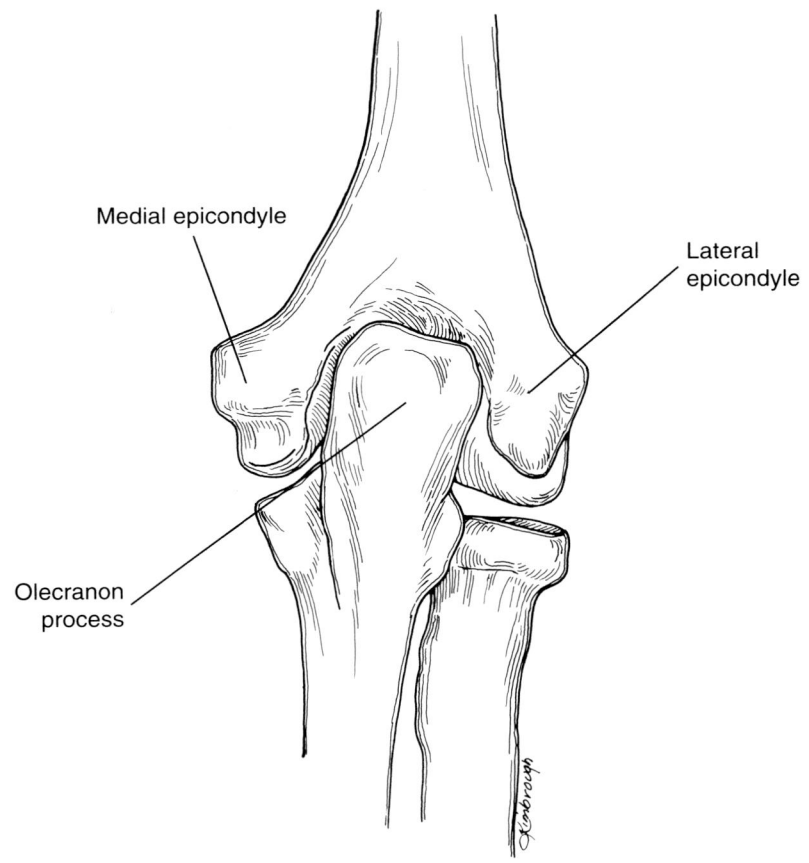

FIG 3–3. Bony anatomy of posterior aspect of elbow.

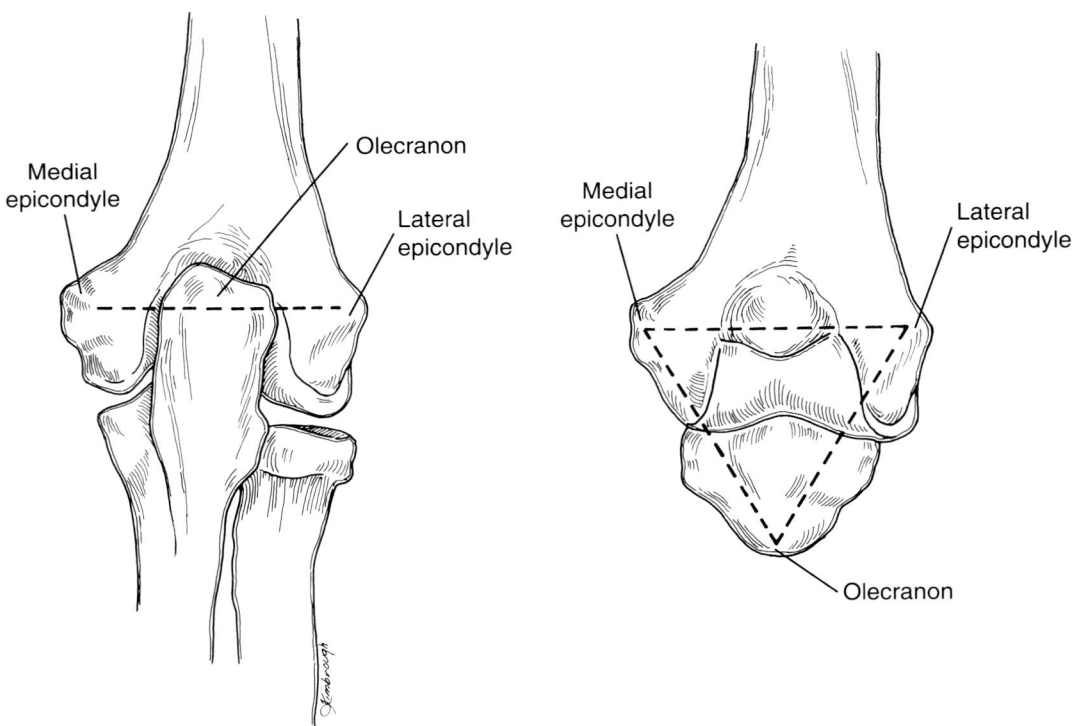

FIG 3–4. Posterior view; medial and lateral epicondyles and olecranon form transverse line with elbow in extension (**A**) and form inverted equilateral triangle with elbow flexed to 90 degrees (**B**).

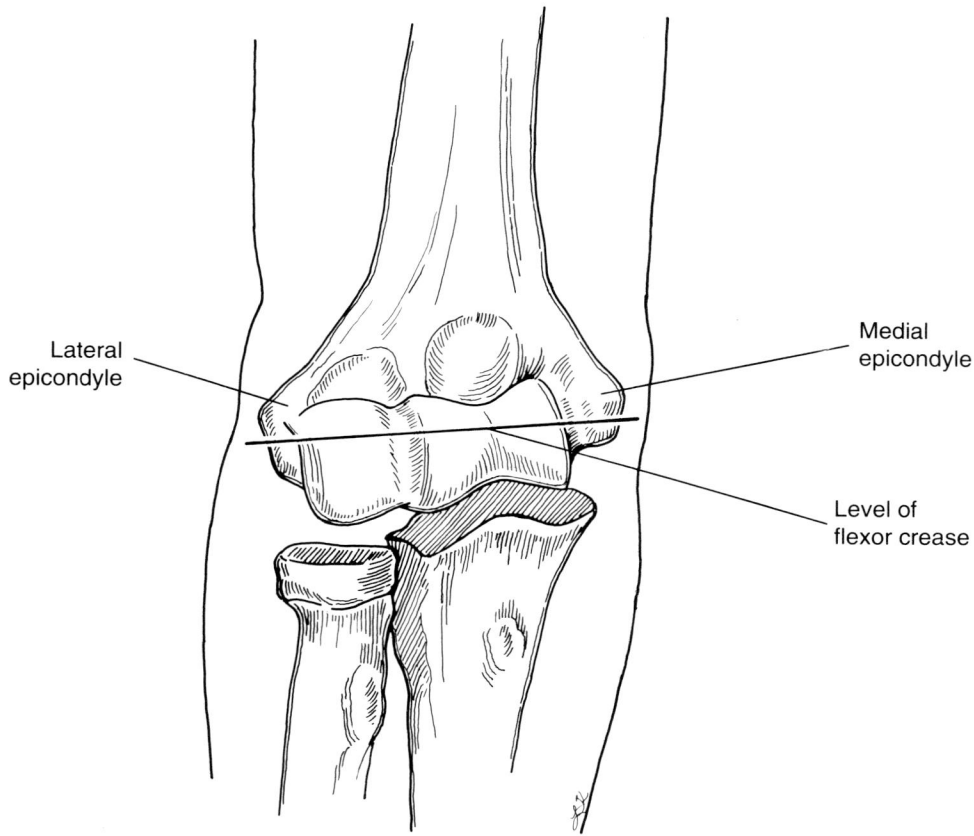

FIG 3–5. Anterior view; level of flexion crease of elbow approximates a line joining medial and lateral epicondyles. Center of elbow joint lies 1 cm distal to this line in the anterior midline.

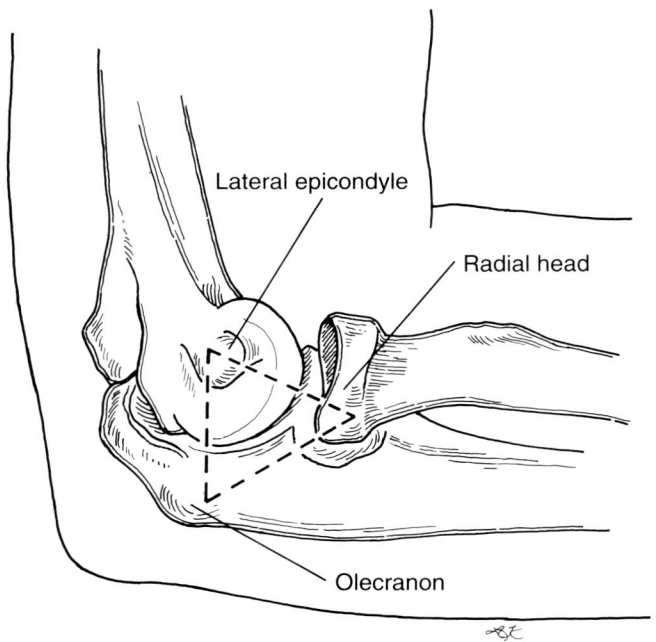

FIG 3–6. Lateral view; lateral epicondyle, olecranon, and radial head form a second triangle, the soft spot.

Intraarticular Bony Anatomy

The distal humerus flares to form its articulating surfaces, which project 30 degrees anterior to the axis of the shaft. The pulley-shaped medial condyle or trochlea (Fig 3–7) is slightly helical, and covered on approximately 300 degrees of its surface by articular cartilage 1 to 2 mm thick. Immediately proximal to the trochlea anteriorly lies the coronoid fossa, which accepts the coronoid process of the ulna during full flexion. The lateral condyle or capitellum is hemispheric and predominantly faces anteriorly. The radial fossa is located just proximal to the capitellum and accepts the radial head during full flexion. On the posterior aspect of the humerus, the large olecranon fossa is located just proximal to the trochlea and is filled with the olecranon process of the ulna during full extension (Fig 3–8). The groove or sulcus just medial to the trochlea guides the ulnar nerve around the posteromedial aspect of the elbow.

The proximal ulna contains a large portion of the joint surface of the elbow. The trochlear notch (greater sigmoid notch, greater semilunar notch, incisura semilunaris; Fig 3–9) of the ulna is a hemicircular ridge formed by four articular facets, of which the two proximal and two distal blend during development.[11] A bare area devoid of articular cartilage normally separates the proximal from the distal articular facets at the center of the notch and should not be interpreted as a pathologic finding. The articular surfaces of the olecranon and coronoid processes form the proximal and distal extents of the trochlear notch, respectively. Immediately lateral to the coronoid process lies the radial notch (lesser semilunar notch), which forms an arc of approximately 60 to 80 degrees and articulates with the radial head. The olecranon process serves as the primary site of the

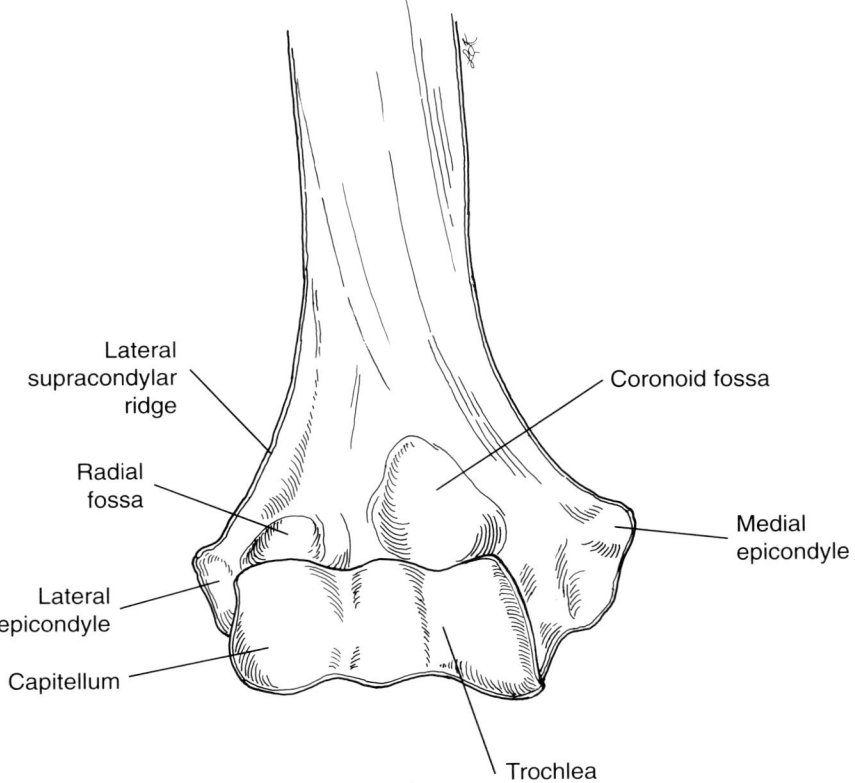

FIG 3–7. Intraarticular anatomy of elbow from anterior aspect. Trochlea is helical and almost entirely covered by articular cartilage.

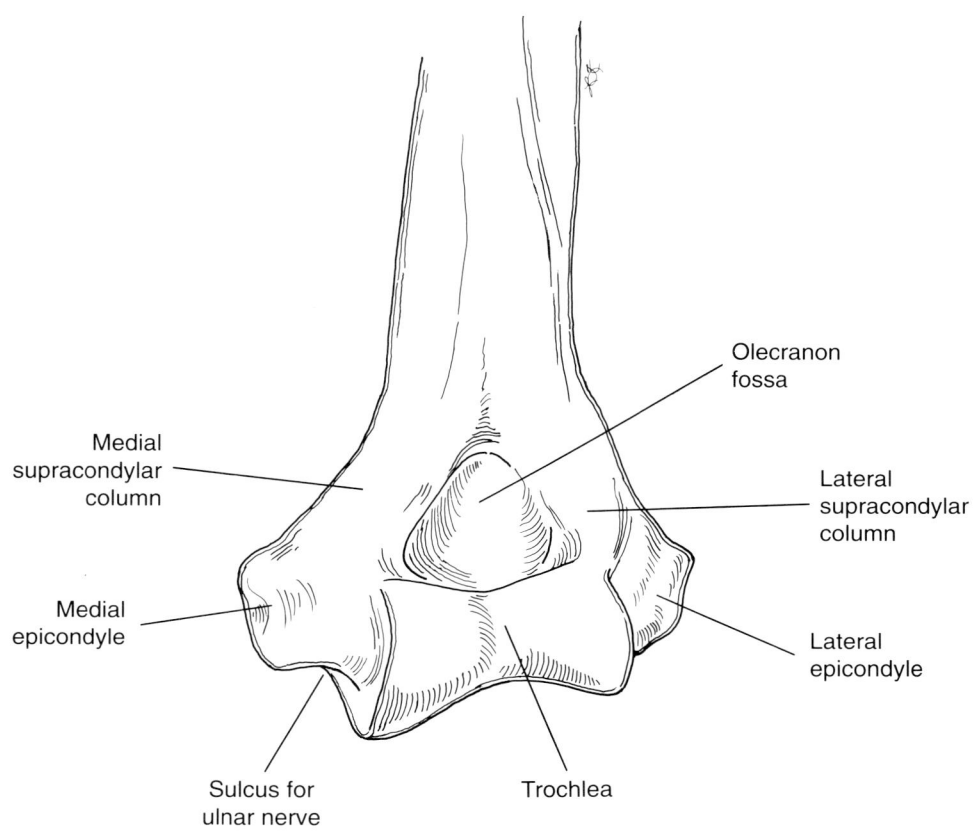

FIG 3–8. Intraarticular anatomy of elbow, from posterior aspect.

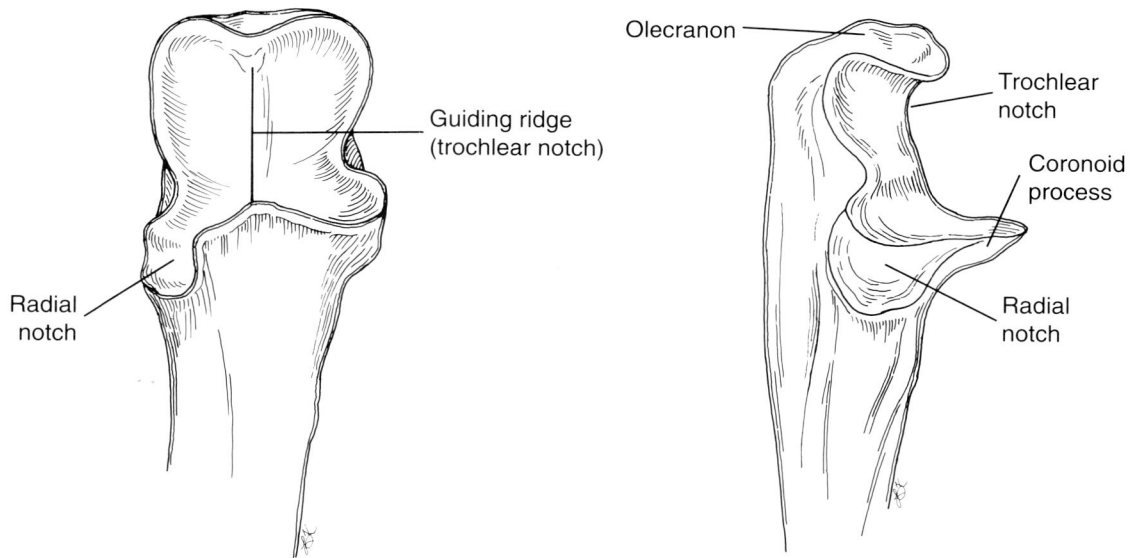

FIG 3–9. Anterior (A) and lateral (B) aspects of proximal ulna.

triceps insertion, and the distal face of the coronoid accepts the insertion of the brachialis muscle.

The head of the proximal radius is mushroom-shaped with a central depression, and except for an arc of 120 degrees on the lateral rim is completely covered by articular cartilage (Fig 3–10). The radial head tapers into the cylindric radial neck. Further distal, the neck blends into the radial tuberosity where the biceps tendon inserts.

The ulnohumeral articulation acts like a hinge (ginglymus joint), and allows 1 degree of freedom of motion, permitting only flexion and extension. The trochlea of the humerus and the trochlear notch of the ulnar mate with great congruency and afford stabiiity to the elbow. Relatively little distraction of this joint is possible. The radiohumeral articulation matches the hemispherical capitellum of the humerus and the radial head and provides for both axial rotation (trochoid motion) and flexion and extension. In the proximal radioulnar joint the radial notch or recess of the ulna captures the radial head, which is allowed to rotate through approximately 80 degrees each of pronation and supination.

The medial collateral ligament complex, which has three components, is the most important of the ligaments that afford stability to the elbow joint (Fig 3–11). The strongest structure is the anterior bundle, which attaches to the inferior aspect of the medial epicondyle and to the base of the medial face of the coronoid process. Portions of the bundle appear to be taut in both flexion and extension. The posterior bundle courses from the medial epicondyle to a broad attachment on the ulna along the medial side of the trochlear notch and is taut primarily during flexion. The transverse ligament lies adjacent to the medial aspect of the trochlear notch and also attaches to the base of the coronoid, but remains entirely on the ulna and offers little support.

The lateral collateral ligament complex is less well defined, but consists of four structures (Fig 3–12). The radial collateral ligament originates from the lateral epicondyle, projects distally to blend into the annular ligament, and is tight throughout the normal range of motion. Funnel-shaped, the annular ligament slings around the radial neck for support during pronation and supination. The lateral ulnar collateral ligament and accessory collateral ligament have been thought to be less important. Recently, the lateral ulnar collateral ligament has been reported to be important in preventing ulnohumeral rotation and posterolateral rotatory instability of the elbow.[12]

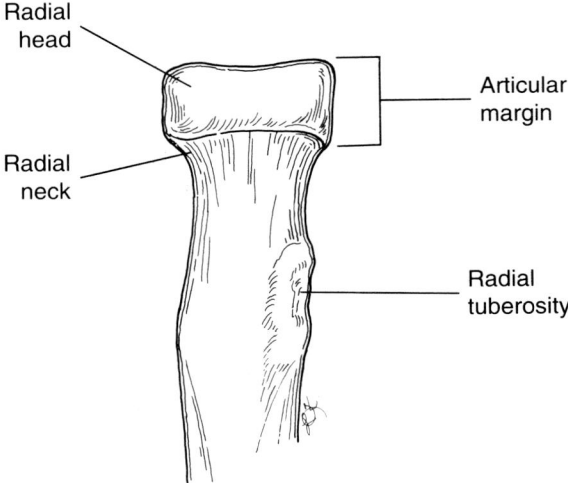

FIG 3–10. Anterior aspect of proximal radius.

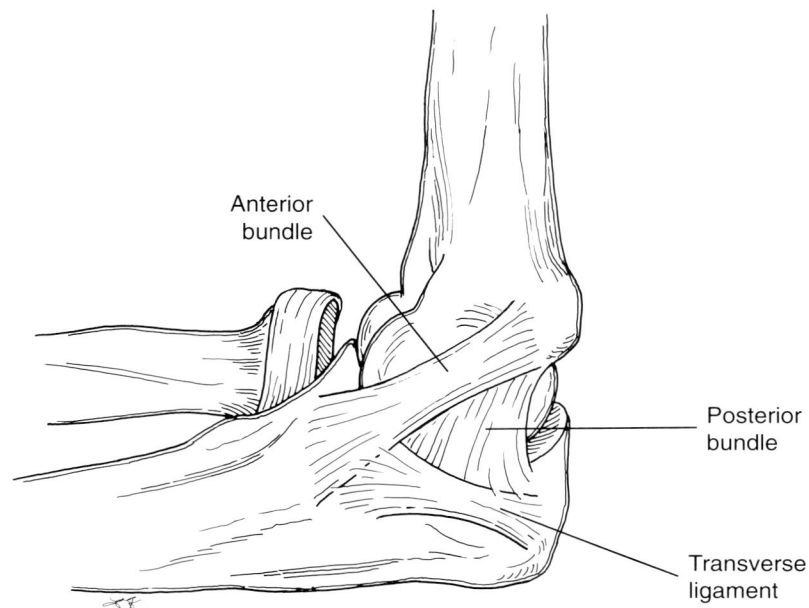

FIG 3–11. Medial collateral ligament complex of elbow.

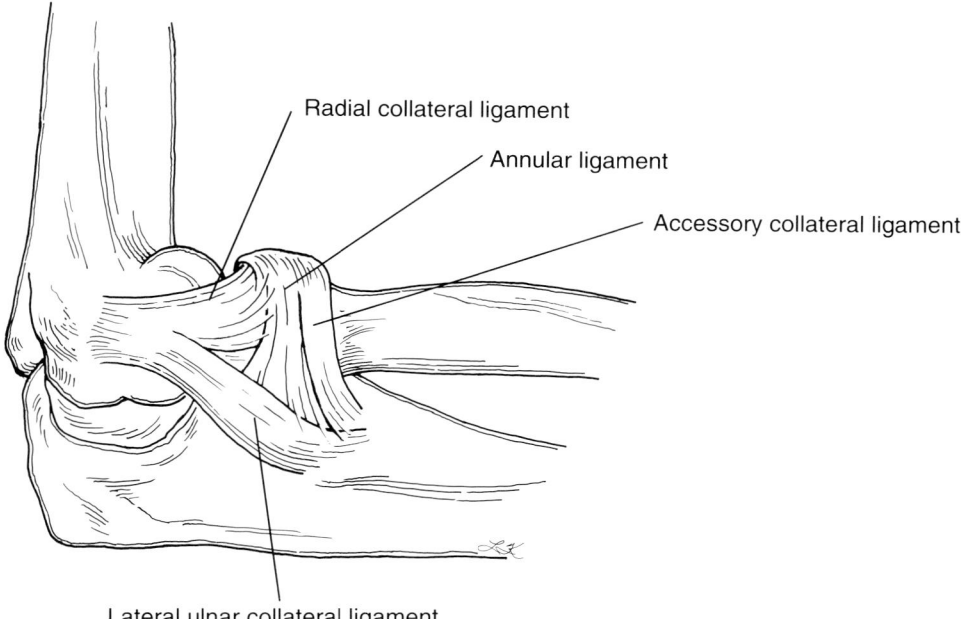

FIG 3–12. Lateral collateral ligament complex of elbow.

Neurovascular Pattern

The cutaneous nerve supply around the elbow derives from various levels of the brachial plexus. The medial brachial cutaneous nerve is a direct branch from the medial cord of the brachial plexus and pierces the deep fascia midway down the arm on the medial side to supply sensation to the posteromedial aspect of the arm to the level of the olecranon. A second cutaneous branch directly from the medial cord is the medial antebrachial cutaneous nerve (Figs 3–13), which surfaces midway down the arm and separates into anterior and posterior branches to innervate the integument on the medial side of the elbow and forearm. After exiting from between the biceps and brachialis muscles, the musculocutaneous nerve gives off the lateral antebrachial cutaneous nerve (Fig 3–14), which divides into anterior and posterior branches to supply the anterolateral aspect of the elbow and lateral half of the forearm. The posterior antebrachial cutaneous nerve (Fig 3–15) branches from the radial nerve, pierces the deep fascia below the deltoid insertion, and courses down the lateral side of the arm to supply the posterolateral aspect of the elbow and posterior surface of the forearm. Although there is some variation, the patterns of the cutaneous nerves are consistent.

The median nerve forms from branches of the medial and lateral cords of the brachial plexus, travels down the arm anteromedially, and courses into the antecubital region on the medial aspect of the brachial artery and biceps tendon (Fig 3–16). As it leaves the antecubital fossa, it disappears between the two heads of the pronator teres and distally beneath the flexor digitorum superficialis. It supplies all of the superficial muscles on the front of the forearm except the flexor carpi ulnaris. Also, the median nerve innervates the majority of the thenar muscles and provides sensation to the palmar surface of the radial three and one-half digits. Assessment of thumb opposition strength and lateral palmar cutaneous sensation are effective tests for distal integrity of the nerve. The anterior

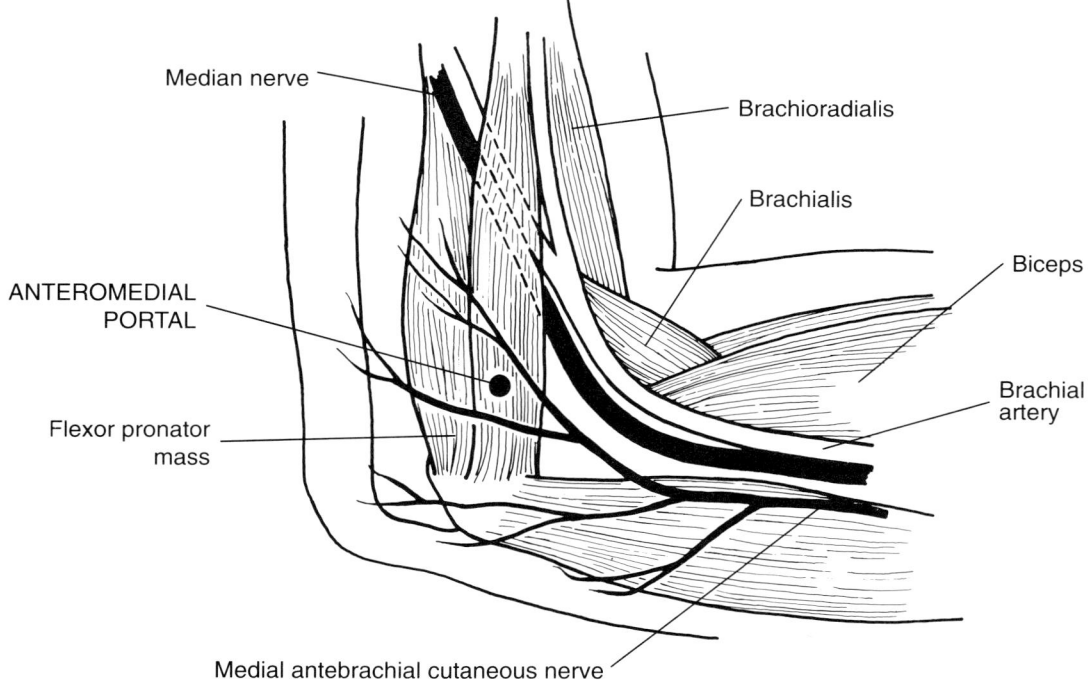

FIG 3–13. Medial antebrachial cutaneous nerve innervates medial aspect of elbow and forearm. (Modified from Lynch GJ, et al: *Arthroscopy* 2:192, 1986.)

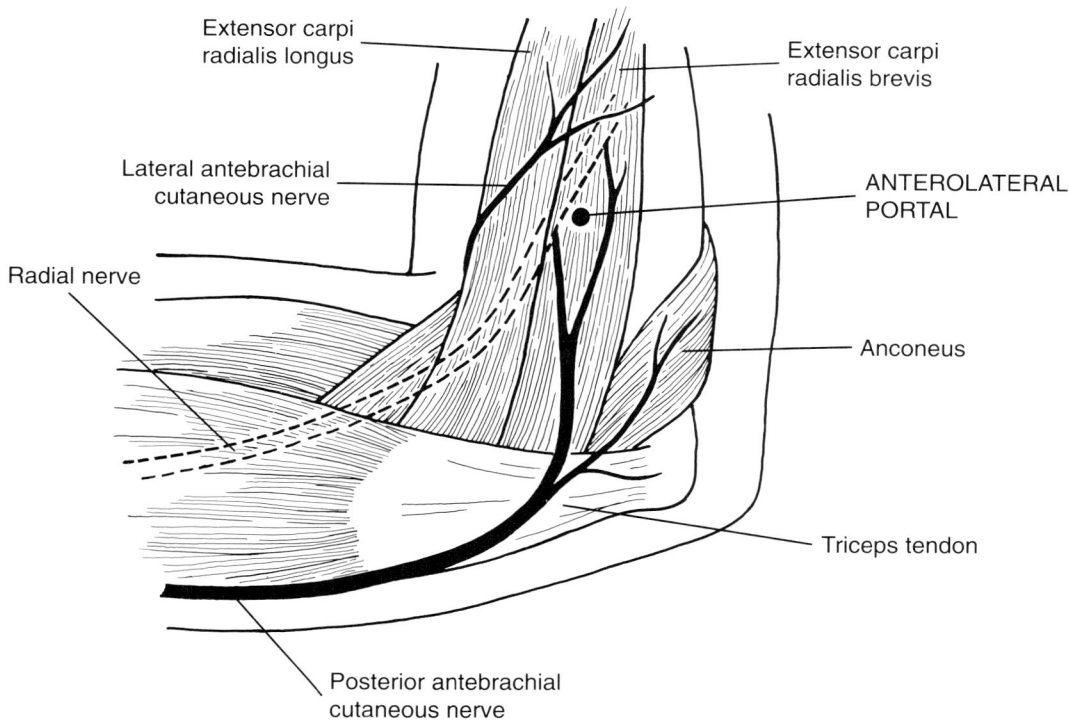

FIG 3–14. Lateral antebrachial cutaneous nerve innervates anterolateral aspect of elbow and lateral aspect of forearm. (Modified from Lynch GJ, et al: *Arthroscopy* 2:192, 1986.)

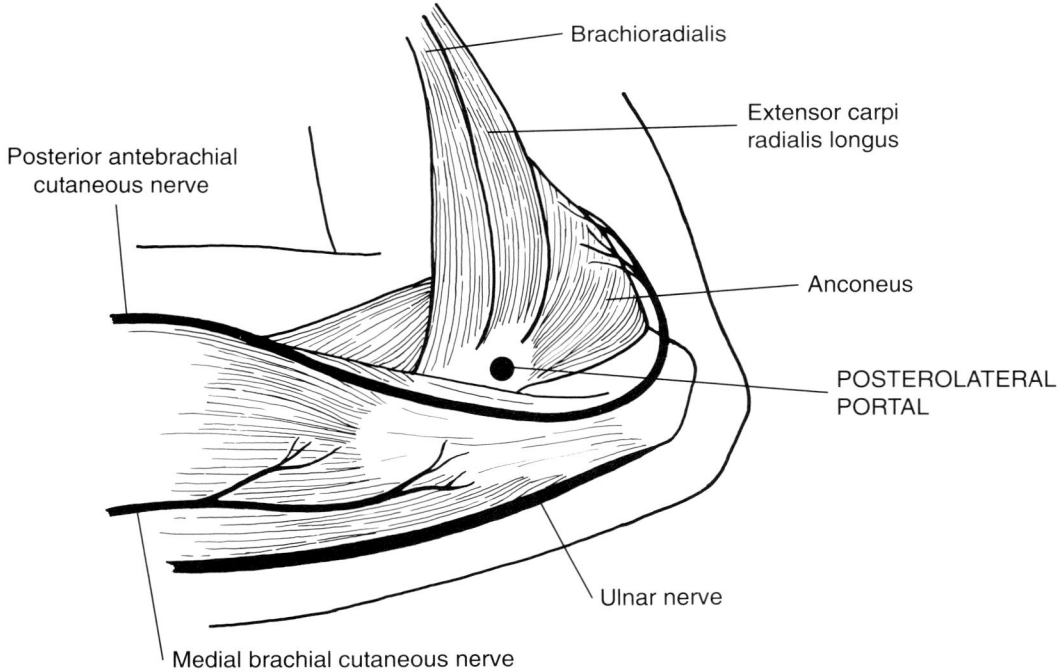

FIG 3–15. Posterior antebrachial cutaneous nerve innervates posterolateral aspect of elbow and posterior portion of forearm. (Modified from Lynch GJ, et al: *Arthroscopy* 2:192, 1986.)

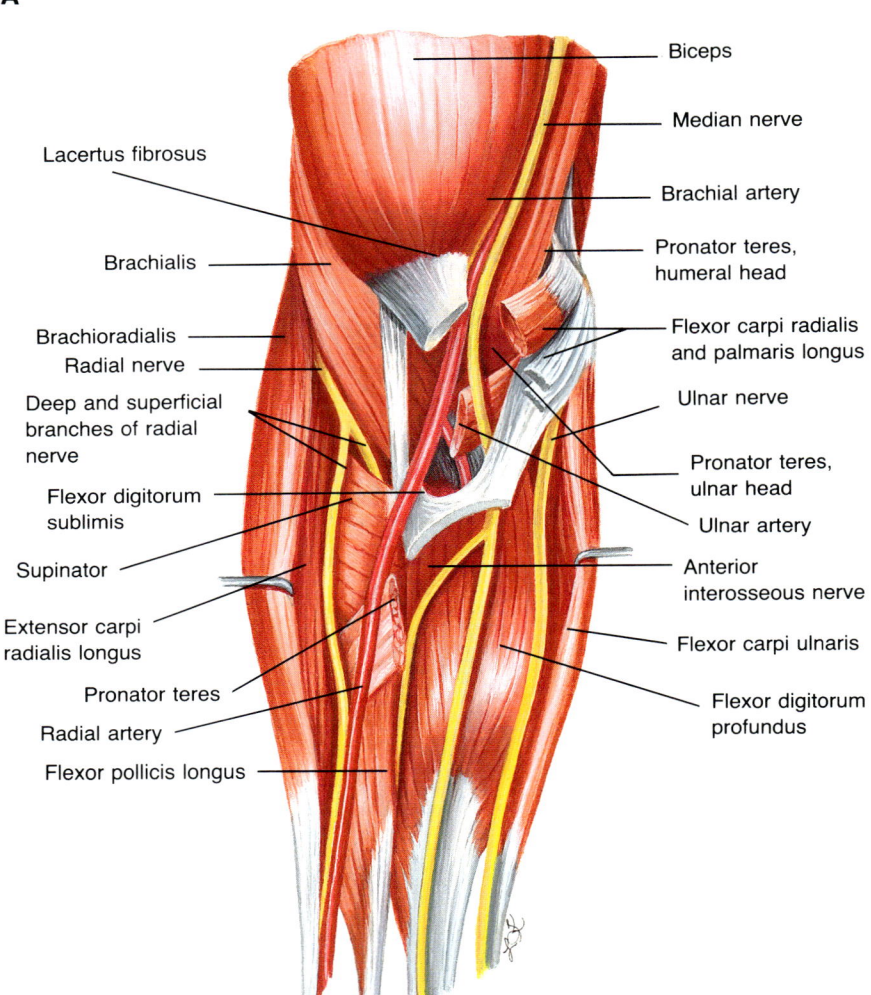

FIG 3–16. (A) Anterior aspect of elbow.

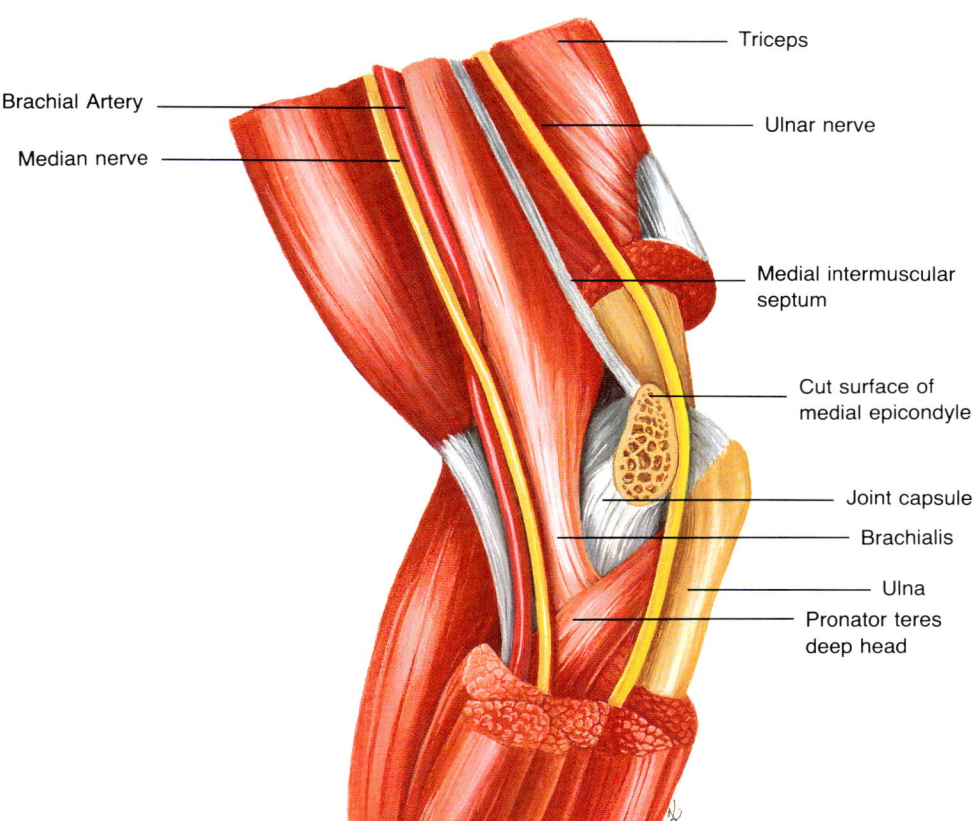

FIG 3–16 (cont.). **(B)** Medial aspect of elbow.

interosseous nerve branches from the median nerve several centimeters distal to the elbow joint. It supplies the deep musculature on the front of the forearm, except the medial half of the flexor digitorum profundus. Loss of motor power for index finger distal interphalangeal flexion implies damage to the anterior interosseous nerve.

The radial nerve (Fig 3–17) is the terminal branch of the posterior cord. It spirals posteriorly around the humeral shaft, and after penetrating the lateral intermuscular septum in the distal third of the arm, descends anterior to the lateral epicondyle between the brachioradialis and brachialis muscles. The nerve divides in the antecubital region. A superficial sensory branch courses distally under cover of the brachioradialis muscle and supplies the skin on the dorsoradial side of the wrist and posterior surface of the lateral three and one-half digits. The other component, a deep branch, wraps around the posterolateral aspect of the radial neck, enters the supinator muscle, and emerges as the posterior interosseous nerve. It supplies all of the muscles on the posterior region of the forearm, which originate distal to the lateral epicondyle. Loss of thumb extension power implies injury to the posterior interosseous nerve.

The ulnar nerve (Fig 3–18) is the terminal branch of the medial cord and penetrates the medial intermuscular septum in the distal third of the arm to reach the posterior aspect. It then courses behind the medial epicondyle, resting on the superficial surface of the

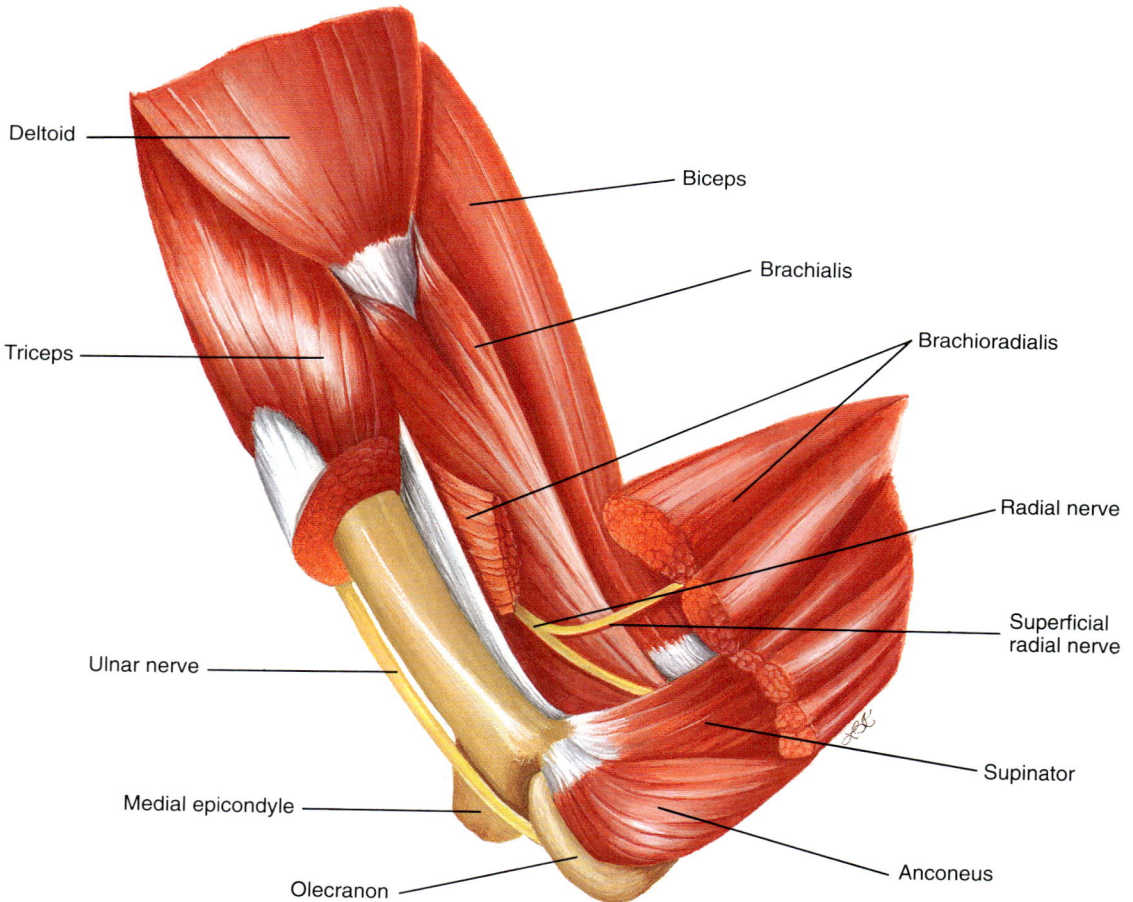

FIG 3–17. Lateral aspect of elbow.

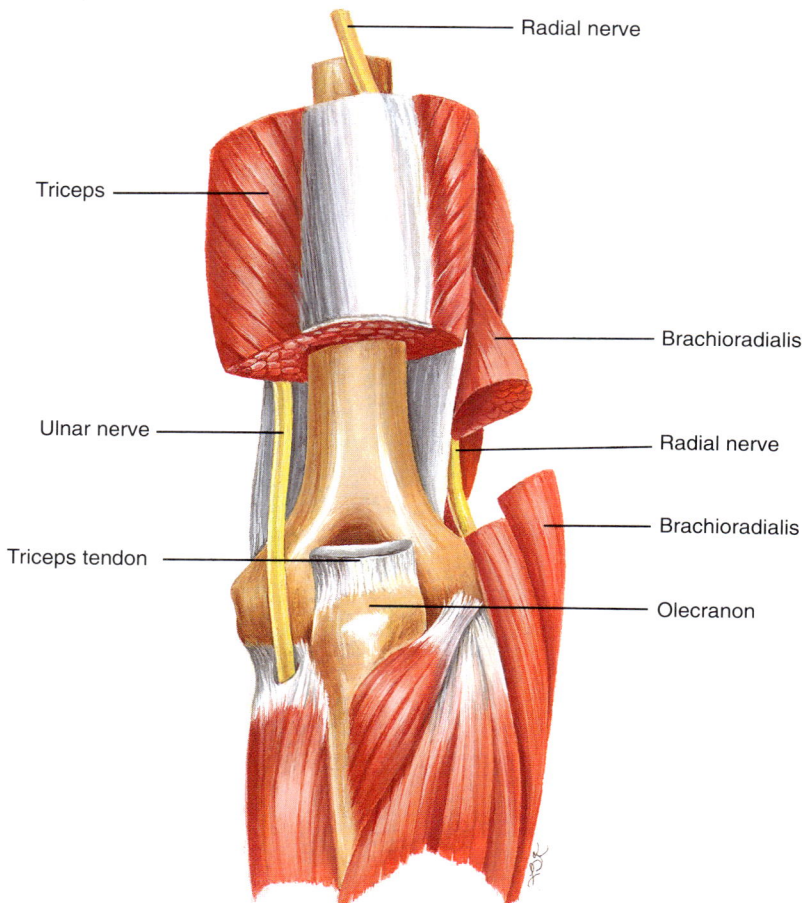

FIG 3–18. Posterior aspect of elbow.

medial collateral ligament. Further distal, it travels between the flexor carpi ulnaris and flexor digitorum superficialis. Although the flexor carpi ulnaris is innervated near the elbow level, no major branches of the ulnar nerve are formed in the cubital region. The muscles of the hypothenar imminence and intrinsic muscles of the hand are supplied, along with sensation for the medial one and one-half digits. Loss of abduction strength of the digits and sensation in the small finger are indicative of ulnar nerve dysfunction.

The brachial artery (see Fig 3–16,A) and several accompanying veins descend into the elbow region on the anterior aspect of the brachialis muscle just medial to the biceps tendon. Approximately at the level of the radial head, the artery bifurcates into its terminal branches, the radial and ulnar arteries. The radial artery passes medial to the biceps tendon before turning anteriorly to lie on the supinator and origin of the pronator teres. In the proximal forearm it lies beneath the brachioradialis muscle. The ulnar artery disappears from the cubital fossa by passing deep to the deep head of the pronator teres, the muscle that separates it from the median nerve. Smaller and somewhat more variable is an extensive system of collateral circulation

PORTAL ANATOMY

The most commonly used portals in elbow arthroscopy include the anterolateral, anteromedial, direct or straight lateral, posterolateral, and straight posterior portals. Several authors have studied the distances of neurovascular structures from these sites (Table 3–1). It is clear that distention of the elbow provides a greater margin of safety in avoiding the deeper neurovascular structures in establishment of the anterior portals.[1] The technique for establishing arthroscopic portals is discussed in Chapter 4.

Anterolateral Portal

The anterolateral portal (see Fig 3–14) courses just anterior and proximal to the palpable radial head.[1] This is usually 2 to 3 cm distal and 1 cm anterior to the lateral humeral epicondyle. This measurement is an estimation of this location and varies in every elbow. Lynch et al[9] determined that this portal is a mean distance of 2 mm from the posterior antebrachial cutaneous nerve. They and Andrews and Carson[1] concur that in the distended elbow the portal passes an average of 7 to 11 mm posterolateral to the radial nerve as it transgresses the extensor carpi radialis brevis muscle and the deep portion of the supinator muscle. Lindenfeld's work,[8] however, indicates that this portal has a much shorter average distance (2.8 mm) from the radial nerve.

Anteromedial Portal

The anteromedial portal (see Fig 3–13) is located approximately 2 cm anterior and 2 cm distal to the medial humeral epicondyle.[1] Several slightly different anteromedial

TABLE 3–1.
Average Portal Distance From Neurovascular Structures*

		Distance (mm)		
Portal	Nerve/Vessel	Andrews and Carson[1]	Lynch et al.[9]	Lindenfeld[8]
Anterolateral	Posterior antebrachial cutaneous nerve	—	2	—
	Radial nerve	7	11	3
Anteromedial	Medial antebrachial cutaneous nerve	—	1†	—
Andrews and Carson[1]‡	Median nerve	6	14	—
	Brachial artery	17	—	—
Lindenfeld[8]§	Median nerve	—	—	23
Poehling[13]‖	Median nerve	—	—	—
Posterolateral	Medial brachial cutaneous nerve	—	20	—
	Posterior antebrachial cutaneous nerve	—	25	—
Straight posterior	Ulnar nerve	20	—	—

*All distances from median, radial, and ulnar nerves are with joint distention.
†Nerve in one of five specimens was cut.
‡Portal 2 cm distal and 2 cm anterior from the medial epicondyle (see text for orientation).
§Portal 1 cm proximal and 1 cm anterior to the medial epicondyle.
‖Portal (patient prone) 2 cm proximal to medial epicondyle, just anterior to intermuscular septum.

portals have been described. Lynch et al[9] found the medial antebrachial cutaneous nerve to be a mean of 1 mm from the anteromedial portal described by Andrews and Carson, and in one of their five fresh cadaveric specimens the nerve was cut during placement of this cannula. When the elbow is distended with fluid and flexed to 90 degrees, this portal passes from 6 to 14 mm posteromedial to the median nerve[1,8] and a mean of 17 mm posteromedial to the brachial artery. The portal courses between the flexor carpi radialis and the flexor digitorum superficialis, then penetrates the deep portion of the pronator teres.

Lindenfeld described a slightly more proximal and posterior entry site for the anteromedial portal[8] than did Andrews and Carson.[1] Lindenfeld's portal is located 1 cm anterior and 1 cm proximal to the medial epicondyle. When the cannula was directed perpendicular to the neurovascular bundle during entry, the average distance from the median nerve was 10.7 mm, and when parallel to the neurovascular bundle, this average distance was 22.3 mm.

Direct Lateral Portal

The direct lateral portal (straight lateral portal, soft spot portal) is in the needle site used in initial distention of the joint, at the center of the triangle formed by the lateral epicondyle, radial head, and olecranon[1] (see Fig 3–16). No neurovascular structures are at significant risk as the cannula passes through the anconeus muscle before entering the joint.

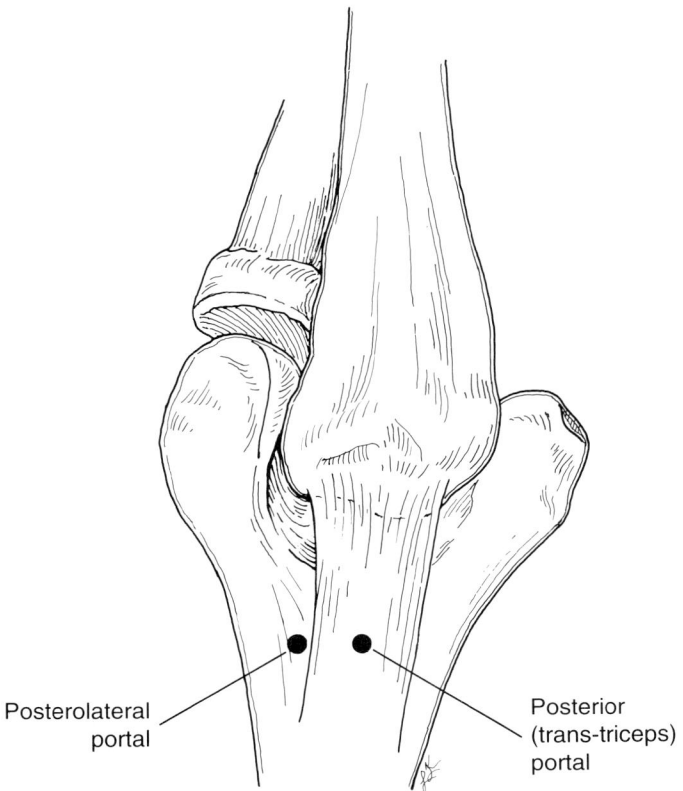

FIG 3–19. Location of posterolateral and straight posterior (transtriceps) portals.

Posterolateral and Straight Posterior Portals

The posterolateral portal (Fig 3–19) is located approximately 3 cm proximal to the tip of the olecranon, just proximal and posterior to the lateral humeral epicondyle at the lateral border of the triceps muscle. The straight posterior or transtriceps portal (see Fig 3–19) is located 2 cm medial to the posterolateral portal, directly over the center of the triceps tendon.

Lynch et al[9] found the medial brachial cutaneous nerve to be on average 25 mm and the posterior antebrachial cutaneous nerve to be on average 25 mm from the posterolateral portal. Provided one does not go medial to the posterior midline, the ulnar nerve remains at least 15 mm from this portal. After penetration of the skin, the cannula will transgress only the edge of the triceps before entering the olecranon fossa.

ARTHROSCOPIC ANATOMY

A detailed knowledge of the anatomic relationships within the elbow joint is particularly important during arthroscopy because any one of the relatively small fields of view may show only a portion of several structures for orientation. The patient may be placed either supine or prone, and although the orientation may be different, the field of view from any particular portal remains essentially the same (Table 3–2).

When the view is from the anterolateral portal (Fig 3–20), the coronoid process at the distal aspect of the trochlear notch is the basic landmark. The majority of the intraarticular portion of the coronoid is covered with cartilage, and a synovial sheath tents the tendinous insertion of the brachialis onto the more distal cortical area. Flexion and extension of the elbow helps to identify the coronoid as it glides in the trough of the trochlea. Adjacent to the proximal articular margin of the trochlea lies the coronoid fossa. Sometimes, capsular thickening in the region of the anterior bundle of the medial collateral ligament is appreciated. As the arthroscope is carefully withdrawn, a small ridge separating the trochlea from the capitellum as well as a small portion of the radial head may be seen.

From the anteromedial portal (Fig 3–21), the radial head is the primary landmark and is obvious as it rotates during pronation and supination. By distracting the radiocapitellar joint 2 to 3 mm, a good view of the central articular depression of the head is possible, for assessment of degenerative changes or depressed fracture fragments. A fold of synovium sometimes projects between the radial head and capitellum, similar to a meniscus. Several authors[3,14] have suggested that this "plica synovialis" may be pathologic. The synovium also reflects over the proximal rim of the annular ligament to form the sacciform recess. Rarely, fibers of the annular ligament itself can be identified. The anterosuperior portion of the capitellum is present in the field of view, as is the bare

TABLE 3–2.

Structures Visualized With Elbow Arthroscopy, by Portal

Portal	Structures visualized
Anterolateral	Medial capsule, coronoid process and brachialis insertion, trochlea, coronoid fossa, radial head (medial aspect)
Anteromedial	Lateral capsule, radial head, capitellum, radial fossa
Posterolateral/ posterior	Olecranon tip, olecranon fossa, posterior trochlea, ulnar collateral ligament (proximal aspect)
Direct (straight) lateral	Radial head, anteroinferior capitellum, trochlear notch, trochlear ridge

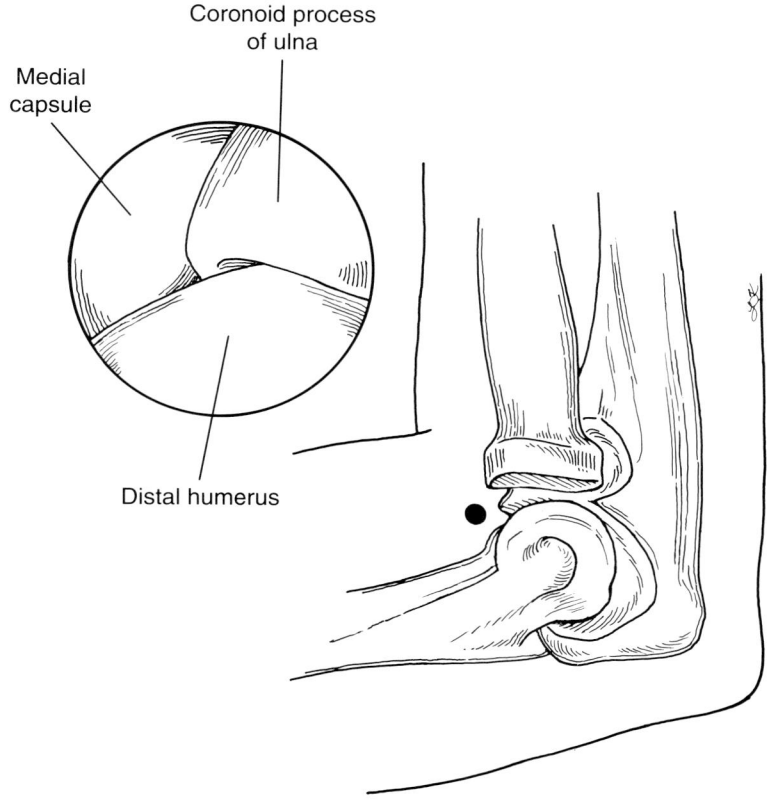

FIG 3–20. *Right*, location of anterolateral portal. *Left*, arthroscopic view from anterolateral portal.

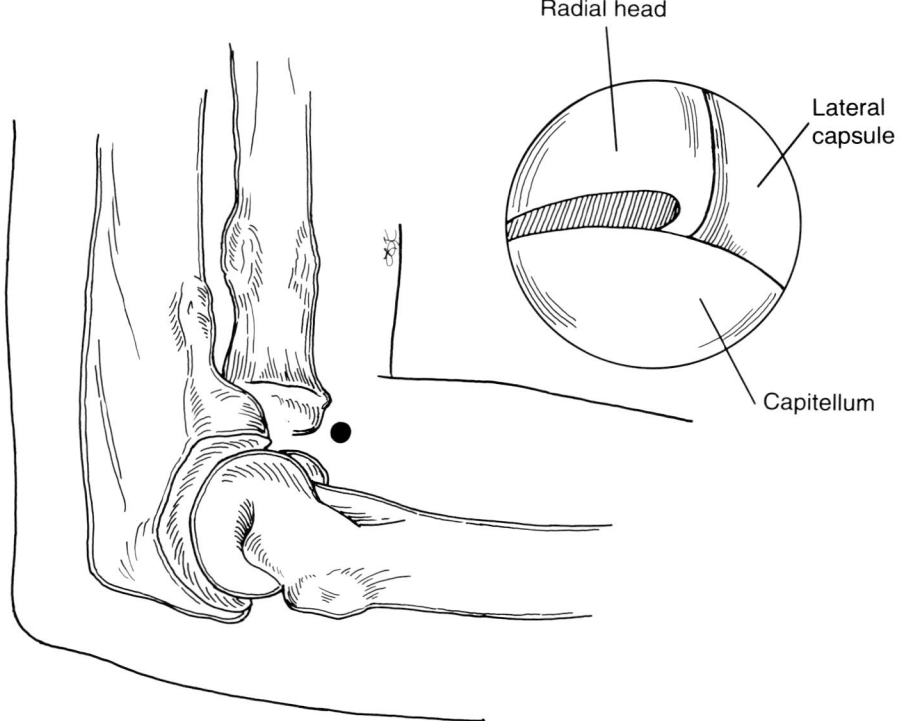

FIG 3–21. *Left*, location of anteromedial portal. *Right*, arthroscopic view from anteromedial portal.

radial fossa immediately proximal to the capitellum. Because the lateral ligamentous tissues are more lax than those on the medial side, a larger harbor for loose bodies is present.

The direct lateral portal (Fig 3–22), or soft spot portal, offers a much greater view of the capitellum when the elbow is flexed to 90 degrees, and osteochondritis dissecans lesions are easily evaluated from this direction. In addition, a more complete view of the radial head is allowed. The trochlear notch may be followed from distal to proximal, and the normal transverse bare area devoid of articular cartilage that separates the proximal and distal facets may be noted.

From the posterolateral and straight posterior portals, the articulation of the olecranon tip with the posterior trochlea is noted during flexion and extension of the elbow (see Figs 3–19 and 3–23). Osteophytes at the posteromedial region of the olecranon and trochlea may be indicative of valgus extension overload.[15] More proximal, the large triangular olecranon fossa may hold loose bodies. In the medial gutter, the ulnar nerve is separated from the bone only by a thin layer of synovium, capsule, and ligamentous tissue, and great care must be exercised in arthroscopy in this area.

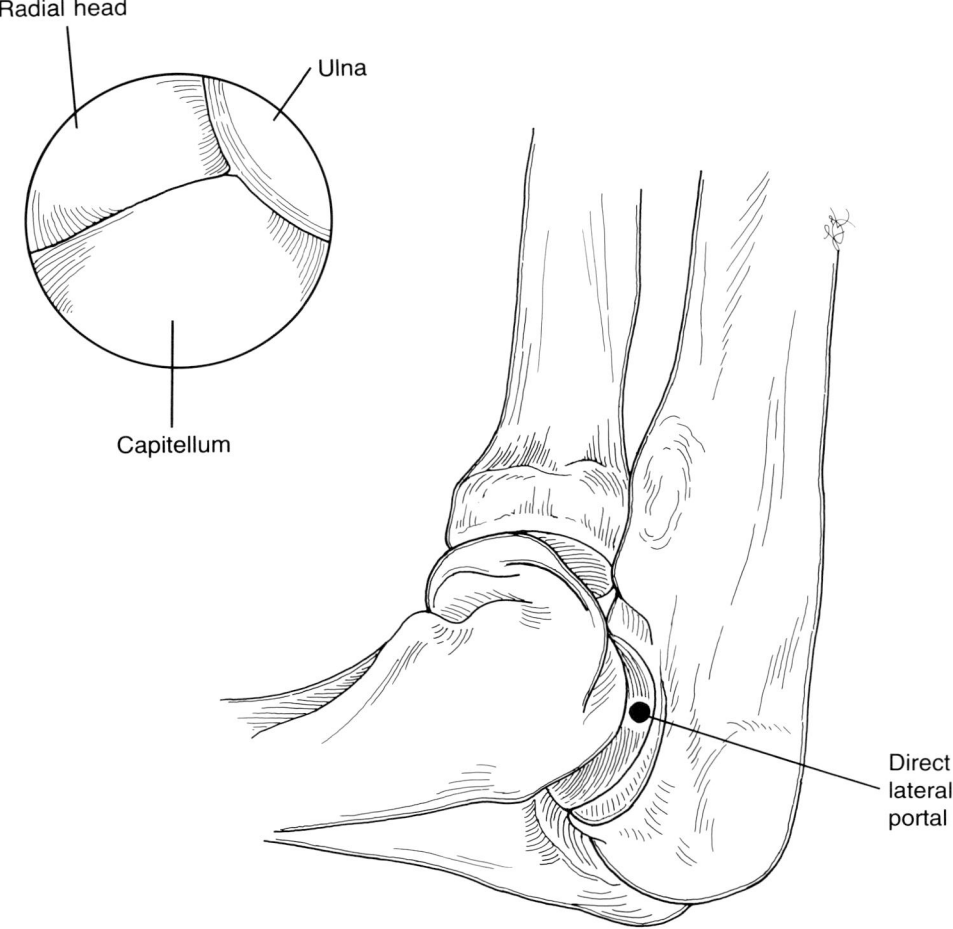

FIG 3–22. *Right,* location of direct lateral portal. *Left,* arthroscopic view from lateral portal.

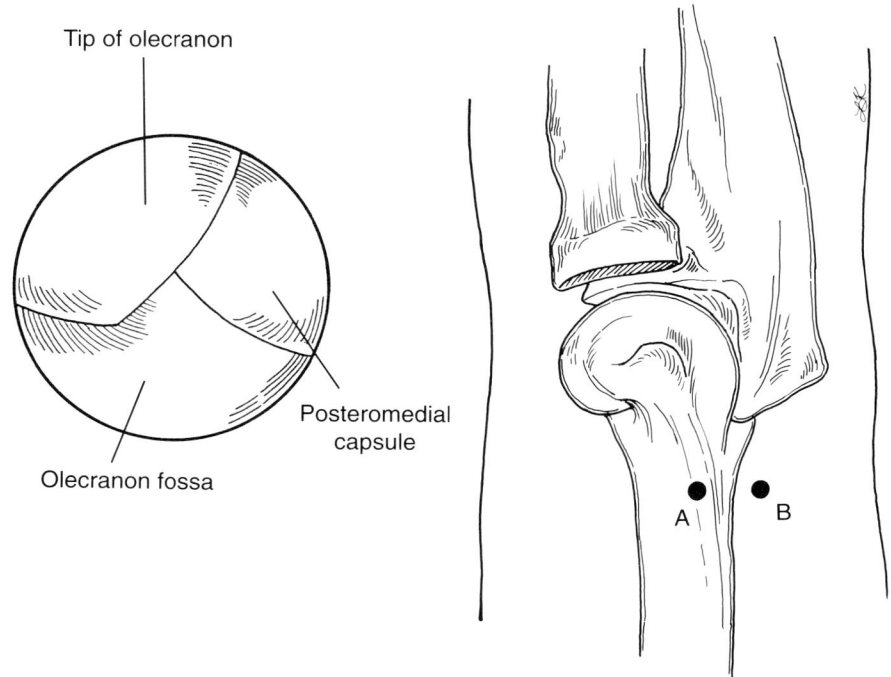

FIG 3–23. *Right*, location of posterolateral *(A)* and straight posterior *(B)* portals. *Left*, arthroscopic view from posterolateral portal.

SUMMARY

To perform elbow arthroscopy safely, a thorough knowledge of regional anatomy is essential. Meticulous attention to detail must be paid to create an accurate map of bony landmarks, and the surgeon should know the proximity of neurovascular structures to the recommended portals. Study of an elbow skeleton to allow familiarization with the bony relationships in the elbow in both the supine and prone orientations from each of the portal views will shorten the time needed for orientation during the procedure and facilitate a more accurate arthroscopic examination. With appropriate preparation, the morbidity of elbow arthroscopy should be low.

REFERENCES

1. Andrews JR, Carson WG: Arthroscopy of the elbow, *Arthroscopy* 1:97–107, 1985.
2. Burman MS: Arthroscopy or the direct visualization of joints, *J Bone Joint Surg* 13:669–695, 1931.
3. Clark RP: Symptomatic, lateral synovial fringe (plica) of the elbow joint, *Arthroscopy* 4:112–116, 1988.
4. Guhl JF: Arthroscopy and arthroscopic surgery of the elbow, *Orthopedics* 8:1290–1296, 1985.
5. Ito K: The arthroscopic anatomy of the elbow joint, *Arthroscopy* 4:2–9, 1979.
6. Ito K: Arthroscopy of the elbow joint: a cadaver study, *Arthroscopy* 5:9–22, 1980.
7. Johnson LL: Elbow arthroscopy. In *Arthroscopic surgery: principles and practice*, St Louis, 1986, Mosby, pp 1446–1477.

8. Lindenfeld TN: Medial approach in elbow arthroscopy, *Am J Sports Med* 18:413–417, 1990.
9. Lynch GJ, Meyers JF, Whipple TL, Caspari RB: Neurovascular anatomy and elbow arthroscopy: inherent risks, *Arthroscopy* 2:191–197, 1986.
10. Maeda Y: Arthroscopy of the elbow joint, *Arthroscopy* 5:5–8, 1980.
11. Morrey BF: Anatomy of the elbow joint. In *The elbow and its disorders*, Philadelphia, 1985, WB Saunders, pp 7–24.
12. O'Driscoll SW, Bell DF, Morrey BF: Posterolateral rotatory instability of the elbow, *J Bone Joint Surg [Am]* 73:440–446, 1991.
13. Poehling GG, Whipple TL, Sisco L, et al: Elbow arthroscopy: a new technique, *Arthroscopy* 5:222–224, 1989.
14. Taillan FA, Comm B, Benezis C, et al: Plica synovialis (synovial fold) of the elbow, *J Sports Med Phys Fit* 28:209–210, 1988.
15. Wilson FD, Andrews JR, Blackburn TA, McCluskey G: Valgus extension overload in the pitching elbow, *Am J Sports Med* 11:83, 1983.

Chapter 4

Diagnostic Arthroscopy of the Elbow

William G. Carson, Jr., M.D.
Stephen R. Soffer, M.D.
James R. Andrews, M.D.

Traditionally, arthroscopy has been most commonly used to evaluate various disorders of the knee joint. Arthroscopy of the elbow is less frequently indicated. In the past few years, it is being used with increased frequency by some arthroscopists, although not by the majority of orthopedic surgeons. It is of interest that arthroscopy of the elbow was first mentioned by Michael Burman[7] in 1931 and that many years passed before arthroscopy of the elbow was once again investigated. More recently, because of technical advances in arthroscopic equipment, development of various arthroscopic techniques for elbow arthroscopy, and our knowledge of the arthroscopic anatomy of the elbow, arthroscopy of the elbow can now be performed on a reasonably routine basis.*

Elbow arthroscopy is a technically demanding surgical procedure, and attention to detail is essential, particularly with regard to the location of the neurovascular structures. Multiple complications of elbow arthroscopy have been reported[13, 14, 28, 32, 33]; many of these complications, however, can be avoided by adhering to a strict surgical technique.

INSTRUMENTATION

Surgical techniques for elbow arthroscopy do not differ much from those used in other joints, with the exception that greater care must be taken to avoid scuffing or gouging of the articular cartilage, particularly of the distal humerus, radial head, or olecranon. The elbow joint is inherently stable, and there is little room in which to maneuver the various instruments. Elbow arthroscopy should be performed slowly and deliberately, to avoid slippage of the elbow capsule and creation of multiple entries of the various cannulas into the elbow joint and resultant fluid extravasation.[8]

Basic elbow arthroscopic equipment includes:

- 18-gauge spinal needles
- Marking pen
- 50-ml syringe
- Intravenous connecting tube

*References 1, 6, 12, 22, 30, 36.

- No. 11 knife blade
- Hemostat
- Hook probe
- Punches
- Graspers with teeth
- Ruler
- Blunt and sharp trocars
- 4-mm 30-degree angled arthroscope
- 2.7-mm 30-degree angled arthroscope
- Interchangeable cannula systems for 4- and 2.7-mm arthroscopes
- Pump system (optional)
- Motorized shavers, trimmers, and burrs

Handheld instruments such as probes, grasping forceps, and punches are commonly used in elbow arthroscopy. Motorized instruments include synovial resectors, trimmers, cutters, and abraders. The use of motorized instruments inserted through cannulas is safer because repeated passes are avoided. Repeated passes create multiple capsular holes and increase the extravasation of fluid about the elbow, thus increasing the risk of damage to nearby neurovascular structures. Whether handheld or motorized, all instruments should be used carefully within the elbow. The instruments should not be wedged between articular cartilage surfaces, because of the possibility that this would cause damage to the articular cartilage. As with any arthroscopic procedure, the instruments should always be in full view.

The arthroscopic systems used in the larger joints such as the shoulder and knee are also used in the elbow. A 4-mm 30-degree angled arthroscope provides optimal visualization of the elbow. Smaller arthroscopes may be used as well. A "small joint system" arthroscopic setup is helpful in visualization of smaller spaces within the elbow, such as the lateral compartment as seen through the direct lateral portal. The overall field of view, however, is somewhat narrower in these small joint systems, and more optimal visualization can be performed with the larger 4-mm arthroscope.

ANESTHESIA

General anesthesia is commonly used for arthroscopy of the elbow because it affords complete comfort for the patient and provides total muscle relaxation. Intrascalene or axillary blocks can also be used; however, some practitioners believe their use requires considerable expertise and increases the difficulty of immediate postoperative neurovascular evaluation. Ito[21] has advocated the use of local anesthesia for diagnostic arthroscopy. Intravenous regional anesthesia may also be used; the use of dual tourniquets about the upper arm, however, can compromise elbow exposure and cause vascular engorgement and edema, thus compromising visualization of the joint.

ANDREWS' SURGICAL TECHNIQUE

A properly padded tourniquet is placed as high on the upper arm and as near the axilla as possible. When tourniquet control is used, care should be taken to use an appropriate size cuff and underlying padding and to limit tourniquet time to no more than 90 minutes. Others claim 120 minutes to be safe.[31]

The patient is placed in the supine position. The hand and forearm are connected to a prefabricated forearm and wrist gauntlet connected to an overhead suspension device, so that the arm is abducted 90 degrees and the elbow is flexed to 90 degrees (Fig 4-1). Five pounds of traction is applied to the arm through a pulley and weight system suspending the arm and keeping the elbow flexed to 90 degrees. This position provides ready access to both medial and lateral aspects of the elbow. The forearm may also be freely pronated and supinated throughout the surgical procedure. At times, the use of an overhead traction device can make the forearm somewhat unstable as it swings on the traction apparatus,

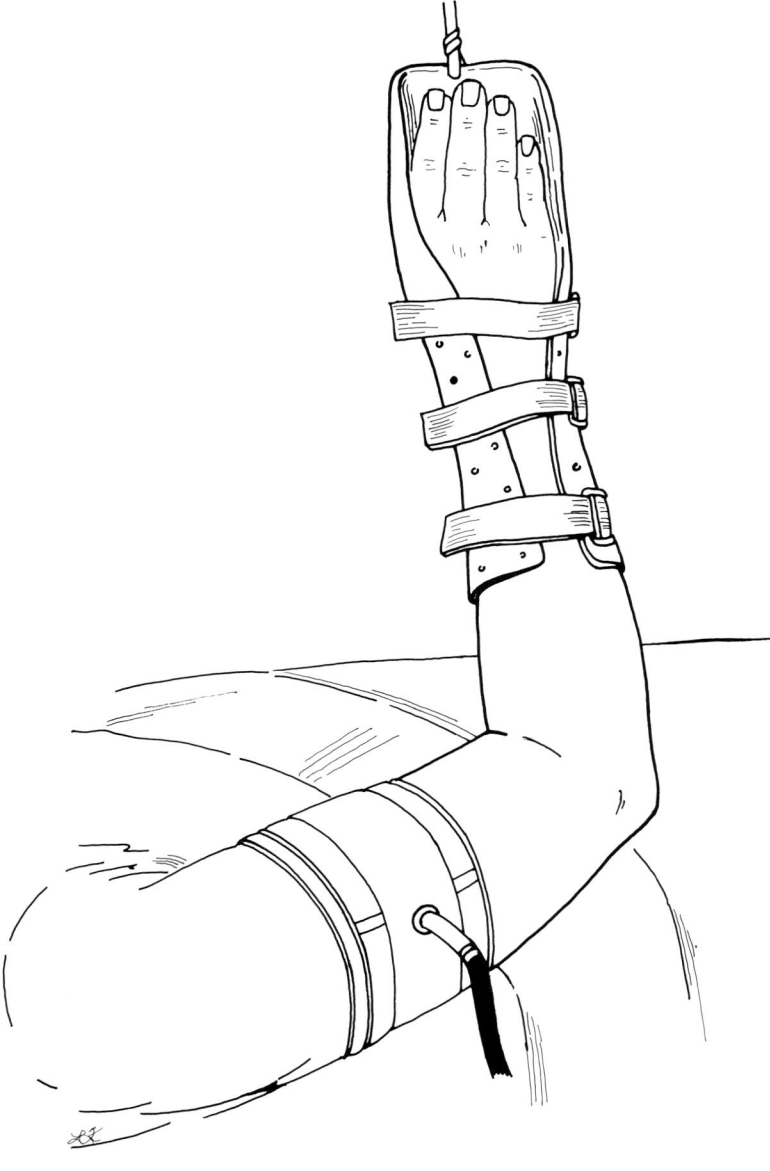

FIG 4-1. With the arm abducted 90 degrees and the elbow flexed to 90 degrees, the hand and forearm are placed in a prefabricated forearm and wrist gauntlet that is connected to an overhead suspension device.

and an alternative to the overhead suspension device is to place two routine operating table arm boards on the same side of the operating table and to allow the arm to rest on this support. With this arrangement, an assistant keeps the elbow in 90 degrees of flexion at all times; this is somewhat more stable than that supplied by the overhead traction device. Whether an arm board support or an overhead traction device is used, the elbow must remain in this 90-degree flexed position at all times when the anterior structures of the elbow are examined arthroscopically, to maintain complete relaxation of the neurovascular structures in the antecubital fossa.[1-11, 26, 27] O'Driscoll et al[27] demonstrated that the intraarticular pressure of the elbow was lowest at 80 degrees of flexion, and capsular rupture occurs at relatively low intraarticular pressure. Rupture of the capsule could lead to extravasation of fluid about the elbow, compromising visualization and making the procedure technically more difficult; thus the flexed position of the elbow should be maintained at all times.

Drapes are used on the upper arm and the patient. A single sterile towel covered by a transparent plastic drape is used to cover the forearm gauntlet. The surgeon sits on the radial side of the elbow, and the first assistant on the axilla side. A Mayo stand can be placed at the end of the table, and the second assistant or scrub technician may stand behind it. Video equipment is placed opposite the patient (Fig 4–2).

After anesthesia has been administered and the position of the patient is stabilized, the bony landmarks are outlined with a marking pen prior to initiation of the procedure

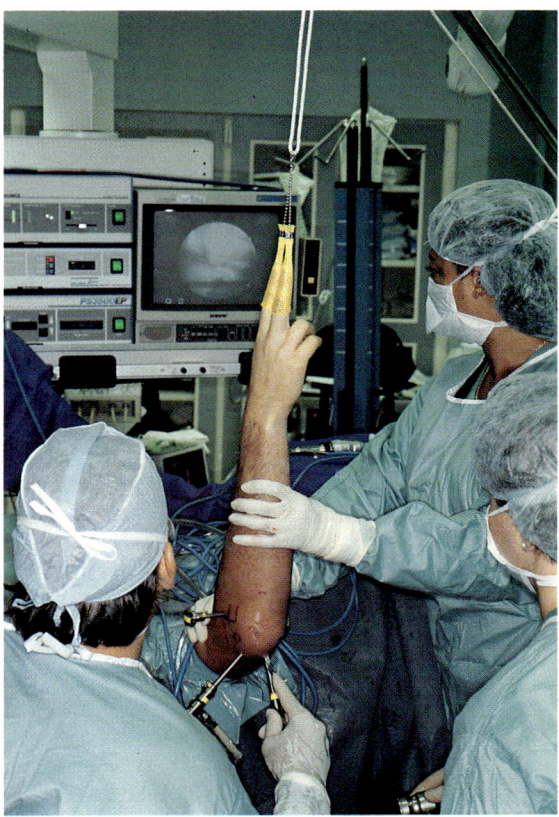

FIG 4–2. Video monitor and other arthroscopic equipment are placed opposite the patient during performance of elbow arthroscopy.

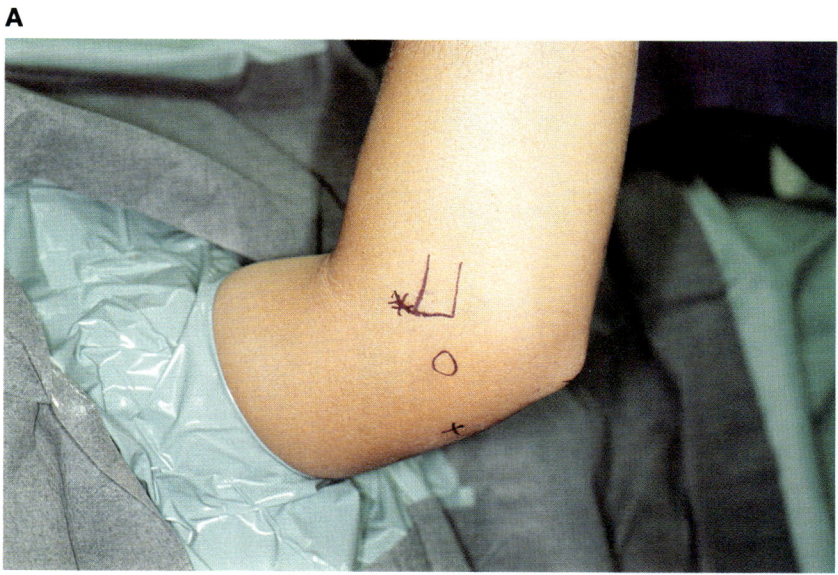

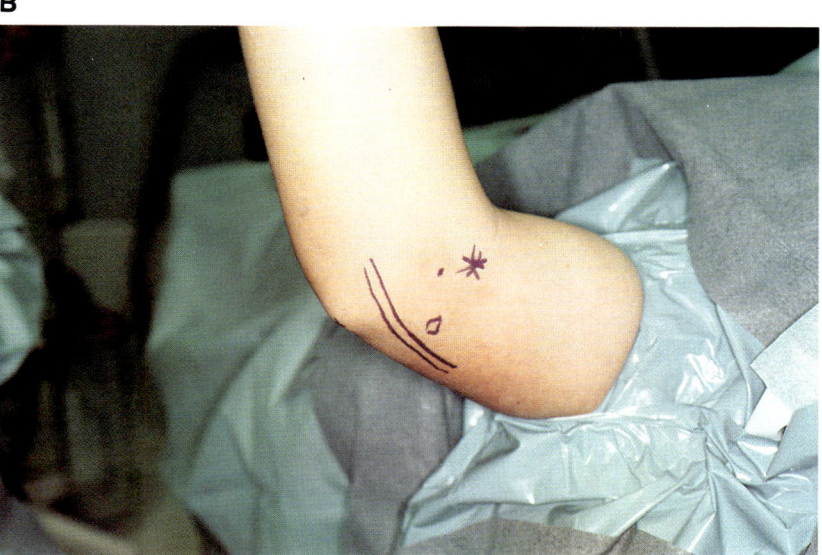

FIG 4–3. Marking pen is used to identify bony landmarks prior to initiation of the surgical procedure. **A,** lateral aspect of elbow. **B,** medial aspect of elbow.

(Fig 4–3). Because large amounts of fluid can be extravasated during the arthroscopic procedure, marking of the landmarks facilitates their identification during surgery. Landmarks commonly marked include the radial head, lateral humeral epicondyle, olecranon tip, medial humeral epicondyle, and ulnar nerve. The anterolateral, anteromedial, direct lateral, accessory lateral, posterolateral, and straight posterior portals are also marked at this time.

The most commonly used portals in elbow arthroscopy are the anterolateral, anteromedial, and posterolateral portals. Other portals have been described for elbow ar-

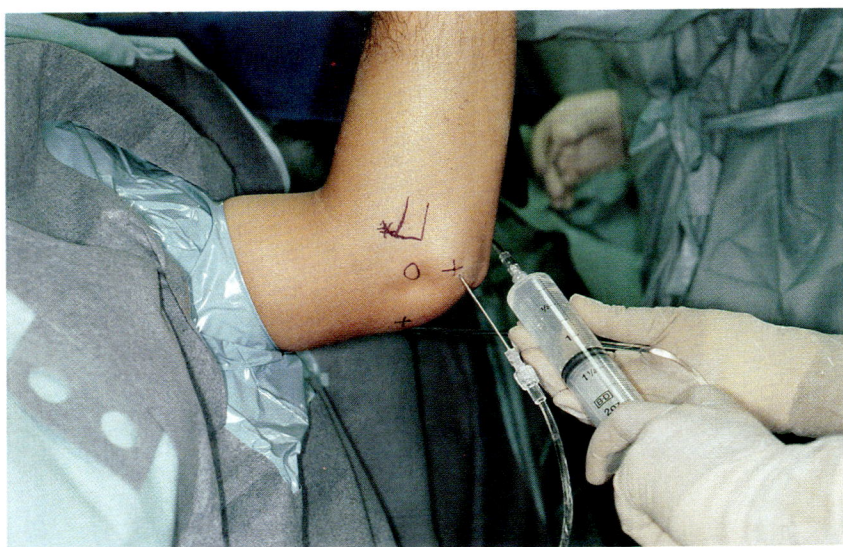

FIG 4–4. Example of 18-gauge spinal needle connected to intravenous tubing and a 50-ml syringe used to distend the joint and as precursor to use of larger arthroscopic instruments.

throscopy,* including several lateral portals[16] and the anteromedial supracondylar or proximal medial portal.[23, 29] In the majority of arthroscopic surgical procedures performed in the elbow, a combination of the anterolateral, anteromedial, direct lateral, and posterolateral portals is used.

Two accessory portals, the accessory lateral portal and the direct posterior or "transtriceps" portal, can be used if required.

Before insertion of the arthroscope into any of these portals, the elbow should be maximally distended with saline solution by using a 50-ml syringe connected to intravenous tubing and an 18-gauge spinal needle (Fig 4–4). The most reliable insertion site for this needle is through the triangular area over the lateral aspect of the elbow, which is bordered by the radial head, the lateral humeral epicondyle, and the tip of the olecranon (Fig 4–5). This is the "soft spot" of the elbow that is often used in aspiration of the elbow as treatment for hemarthrosis. When this area is penetrated, the 18-gauge needle traverses skin, a thin subcutaneous layer, the anconeus muscle, and the capsule. Proper placement into the elbow joint is verified by free backflow from the needle (Fig 4–6). After entry into the elbow is verified and 30 mL saline solution is injected, the needle is removed and the elbow is left maximally distended. At this time the primary diagnostic portal of choice may be established.

Anterolateral Portal

We prefer to use the anterolateral portal as the standard diagnostic portal for arthroscopy of the elbow, and this portal is established first. The landmarks and portals, as mentioned previously, are outlined with a methylene blue sterile marker at the outset of the procedure. To palpate the radial head, one places the index finger or thumb over the radiocapitellar joint line while pronating and supinating the forearm. The entire radial head is outlined with the marker. The point just anterior and proximal to the radial head is marked as the anterolateral portal. This portal is usually 2 to 3 cm distal and 1 cm

*References 15, 18, 19, 20, 22, 25, 35.

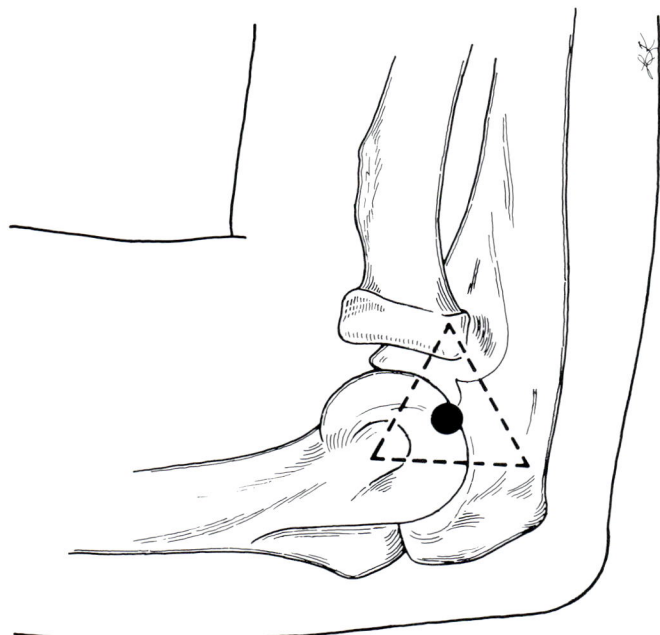

FIG 4–5. Insertion site for the 18-gauge spinal needle for initial distention of the elbow is located through the triangular area bordered by the lateral humeral epicondyle, the radial head, and the tip of the olecranon.

anterior to the lateral humeral epicondyle (Fig 4–7). The key to the location of this portal is that it lies just anterior and proximal to the radial head; the 2 to 3 × 1-cm measurement is an *estimation* of this location and varies in every elbow (Fig 4–8). As described, the elbow is flexed 90 degrees, and an 18-gauge needle is placed in the soft spot. The elbow joint is maximally distended with 30 mL sterile saline solution injected through the 18-

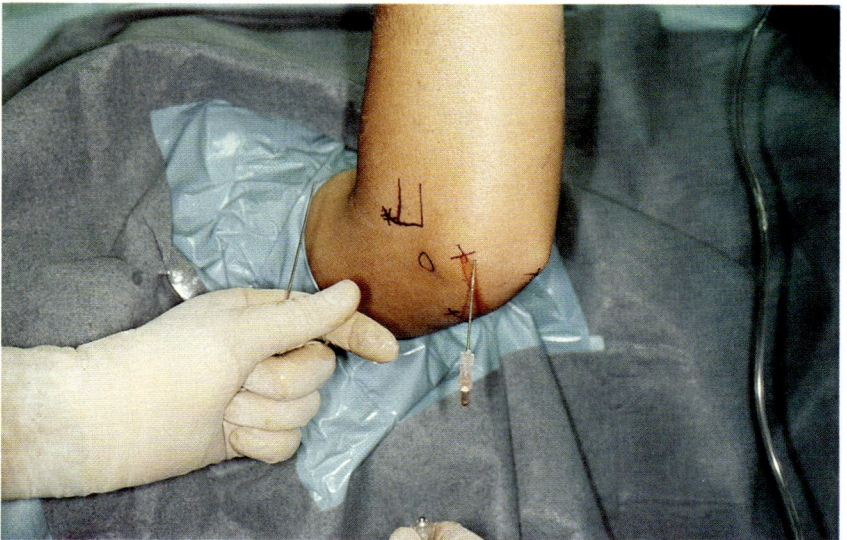

FIG 4–6. Proper placement into the elbow joint is verified by backflow of fluid from the 18-gauge spinal needle.

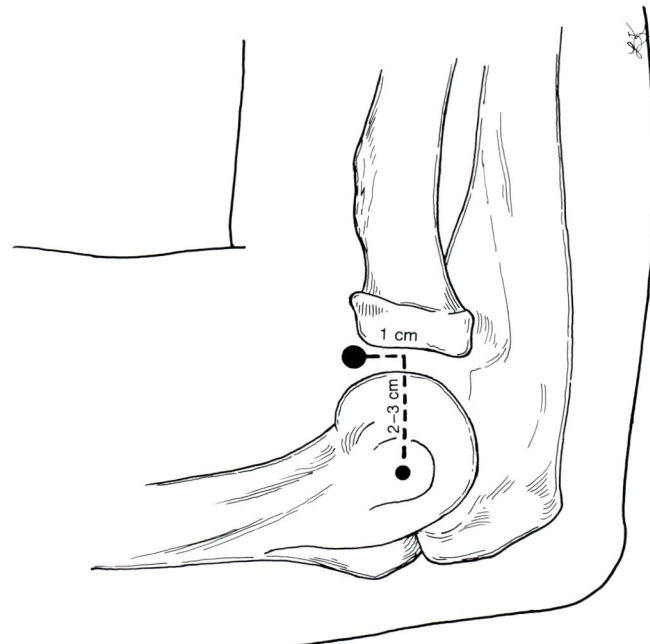

FIG 4–7. Anterolateral portal is located approximately 2 to 3 cm distal and 1 cm anterior to the lateral humeral epicondyle.

gauge spinal needle. After distention is complete, a second 18-gauge spinal needle is placed at the point previously marked as the anterolateral portal. The needle is aimed directly toward the center of the joint. Location of this second needle in the elbow joint is confirmed by free backflow of fluid.

Once proper placement of the 18-gauge needle is confirmed and the elbow is maximally distended and flexed 90 degrees, the larger arthroscopic instruments, such as the

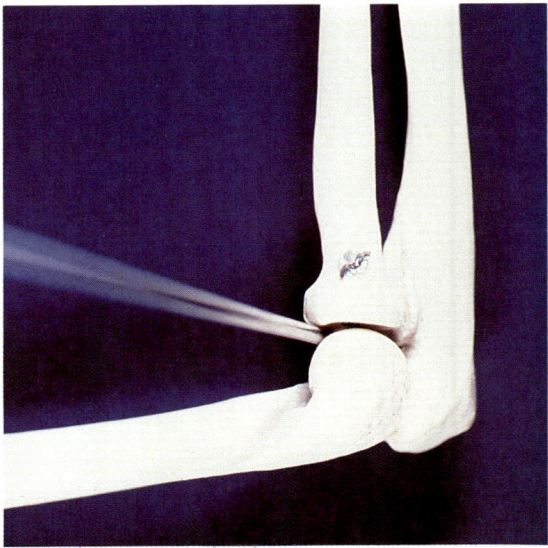

FIG 4–8. Through the anterolateral arthroscopic portal, instruments enter the elbow anterior to the radial head.

arthroscope itself and the cannula system, can be introduced (Fig 4–9). The cannula system is introduced by making a small incision in the skin only, with care to avoid injury to the underlying subcutaneous nerves. Close attention should be given to the subcutaneous nerves about the elbow during establishment of these portals. A No. 11 blade is laid against the skin, and the skin is then pulled across the blade. The incision and the underlying subcutaneous tissues may then be deepened by using a hemostat.[24] The lateral and posterior antebrachial cutaneous nerves must be avoided (Fig 4–10).

At this point, a blunt trocar is used because it can be readily inserted through the subcutaneous fat and muscles. Use of the blunt trocar during insertion of the cannula minimizes damage to nearby neurovascular structures and articular cartilage (Figs 4–10 and 4–11).

Careful attention must be given to the angle of insertion of the trocar and cannula system. The instruments should be directed to the center of the elbow with the elbow flexed at 90 degrees at all times. As the surgeon aims the trocar and cannula toward the joint, the capsule and synovium must be "trapped" against the distal humerus to puncture it and enter the elbow joint (Fig 4–12). Once the capsule is entered, free backflow of fluid through the cannula will be evident, verifying entrance into the elbow. At this time the arthroscope is inserted, and diagnostic arthroscopy is begun.

Continuous distention of the elbow is maintained by using two 3-L bags of normal saline solution elevated above the patient and attached to the arthroscope, allowing distention by way of gravity. An alternative is to use an infusion pump to distend the elbow; this method is used for all elbow arthroscopy by Dr. Andrews, at the American Sports Medicine Institute. One pump system (3M Company, Minneapolis) has been developed to allow pump inflow to run through the arthroscopic cannula and to permit pressure sensing at the tip of the arthroscope. With this system, pressure within the joint is sensed, and an alarm sounds when the pressure exceeds safe boundaries. Maximum pump pressure for elbow arthroscopy should not exceed 50 mm Hg. If an arthroscopic cannula with an outflow sleeve is being used, intermittent suction through this sleeve may be used to remove any cloudy fluid or debris. Unless cleansing is required, the sleeve is usually

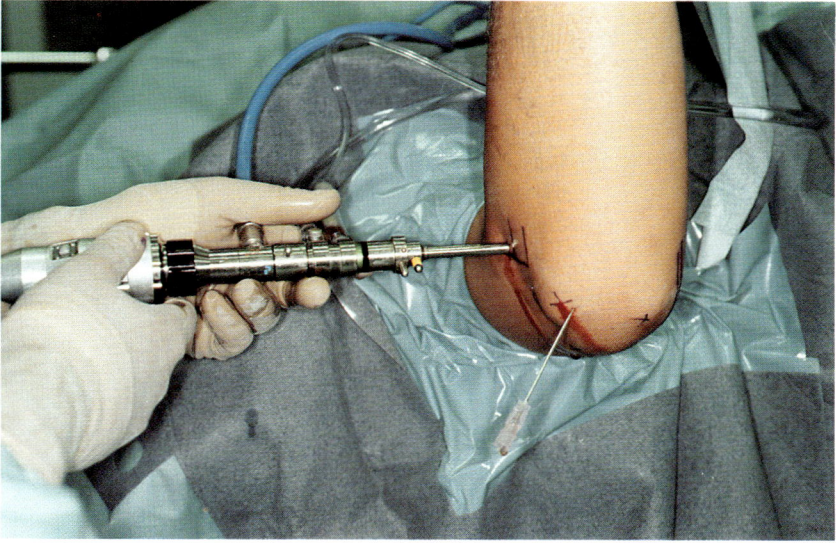

FIG 4–9. Example of 4-mm 30-degree angled arthroscope in place through the anterolateral portal.

42 Chapter 4

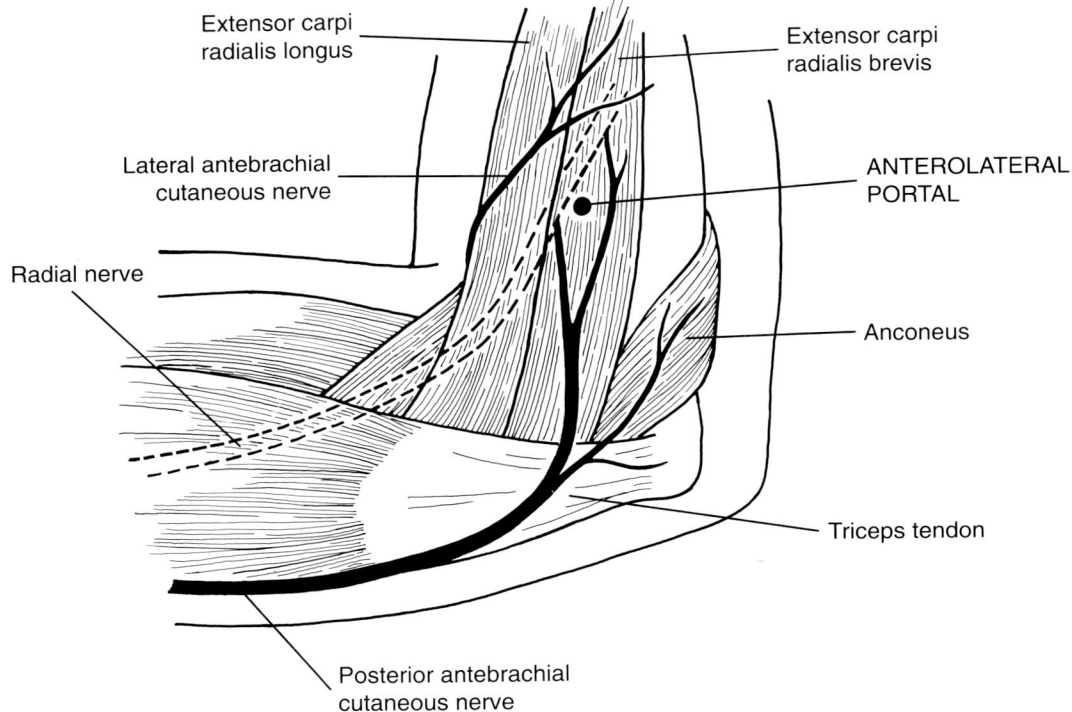

FIG 4–10. Anatomy of the lateral and posterior antebrachial cutaneous nerves. (Modified from Lynch GJ, et al: *Arthroscopy* 2:192, 1986.)

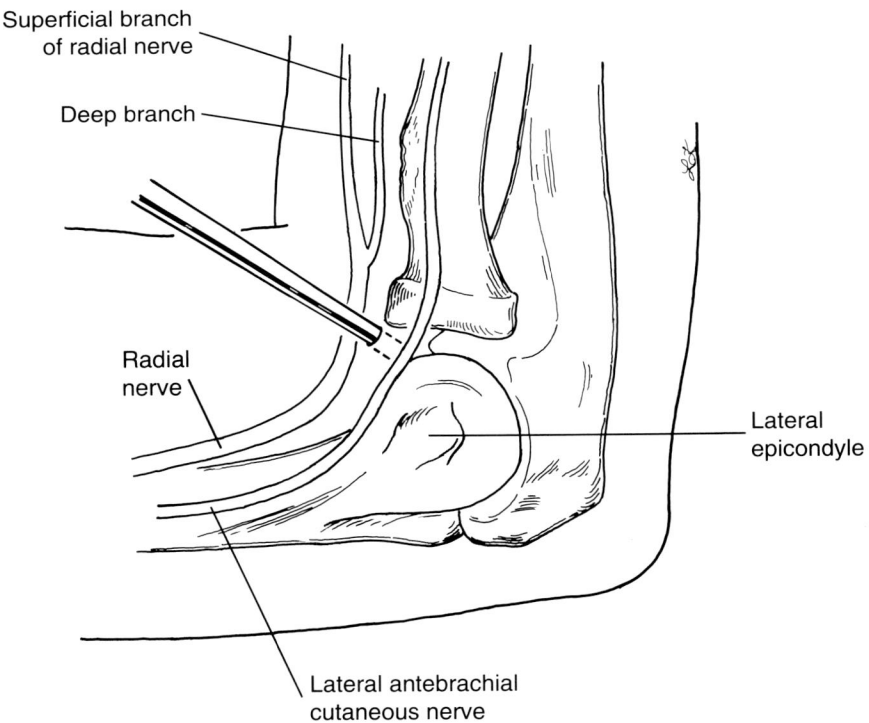

FIG 4–11. Arthroscope courses just anterior to the radial head and passes inferior to the radial nerve.

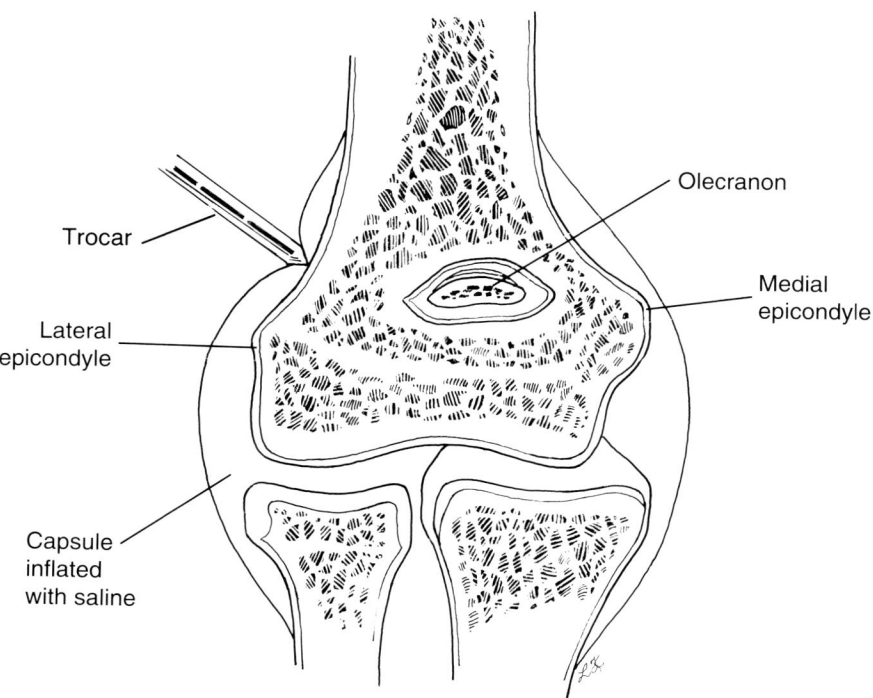

FIG 4–12. Synovium and capsule being trapped against the distal humerus by the trocar and cannula.

left clamped off, to maintain distention pressure within the elbow. During insertion of larger instruments into the elbow joint, it is important that the elbow is kept maximally distended, because this further displaces the neurovascular structures (e.g., the radial nerve laterally and the median nerve medially) away from the entering arthroscopic instruments[24] (see Chapter 7).

Anteromedial Portal

After the anterolateral portal has been established, the anteromedial portal is established by way of direct intraarticular visualization. The anteromedial portal is identified approximately 2 cm anterior and 2 cm distal to the medial humeral epicondyle (Fig 4–13). With the arthroscope in the anterolateral portal, an 18-gauge spinal needle is inserted at the entry point described above, with the elbow flexed 90 degrees. The elbow is maximally distended with the fluid, and the needle is aimed directly toward the center of the joint (Fig 4–14). Confirmation that the needle is entering the joint is provided by direct visualization through the arthroscope in the anterolateral portal. The needle passes just anterior to the medial humeral epicondyle and inferior to the antecubital structures (Figs 4–15 and 4–16). The ideal position of the needle is just proximal to the humeral ulnar joint and just anterior to the humerus. Again, the 2 × 2-cm location mentioned above is an *estimation* of the ideal position of the anteromedial portal and varies in elbows of different sizes.

The stylet may be removed from the spinal needle. This allows a temporary outflow system for air bubbles and debris that may obscure visualization. After these bubbles and debris are cleared, the areas of needle entry should be carefully evaluated, with appropriate adjustments then made if necessary.

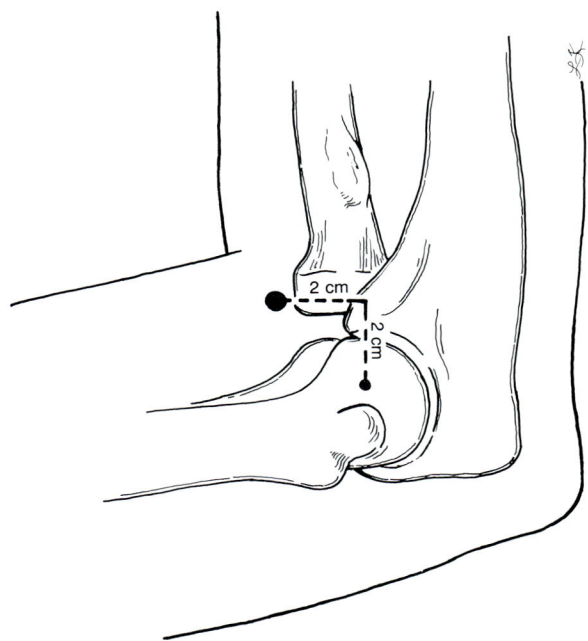

FIG 4–13. Anteromedial portal is located approximately 2 cm anterior and 2 cm distal to the medial humeral epicondyle.

A small incision is made in the skin, with care taken to protect the subcutaneous nerves (see Fig 4–16), and the arthroscopic cannula and blunt trocar system are introduced (Fig 4–17). An interchangeable cannula system is used to change freely from the anterolateral to the anteromedial portal with the various instruments. If a simple diagnostic arthroscopy is being performed, an inflow cannula can be placed through the anteromedial portal to provide better distention and visualization. Because maximum distention of the

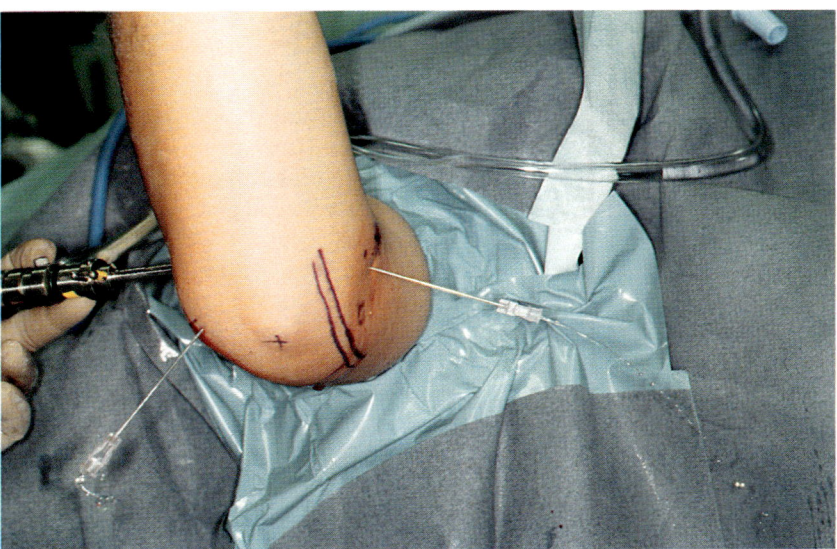

FIG 4–14. With the arthroscope in place in the anterolateral portal, an 18-gauge spinal needle is placed through the anteromedial portal.

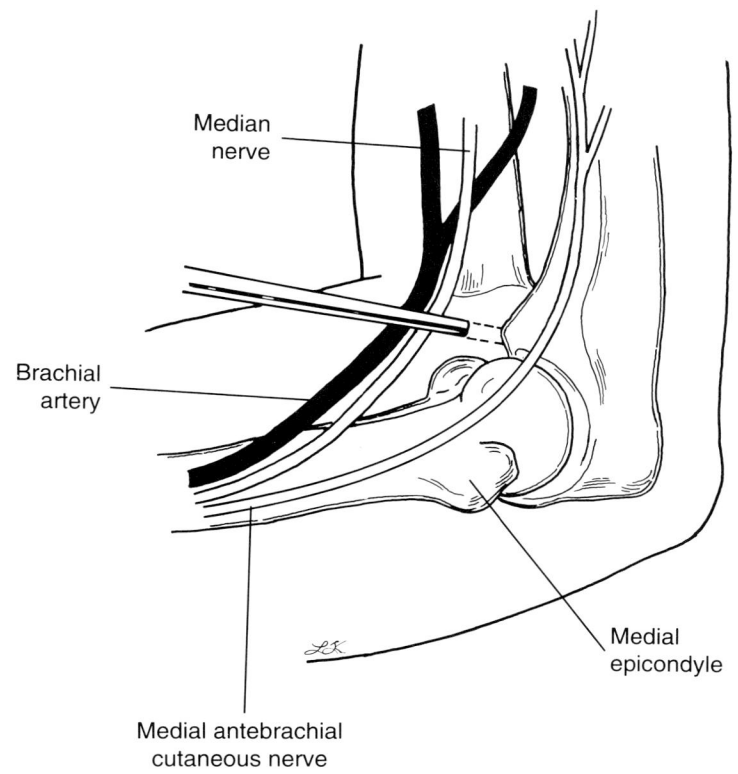

FIG 4–15. Arthroscope passes just anterior to the medial humeral epicondyle and inferior to the median nerve and brachial artery.

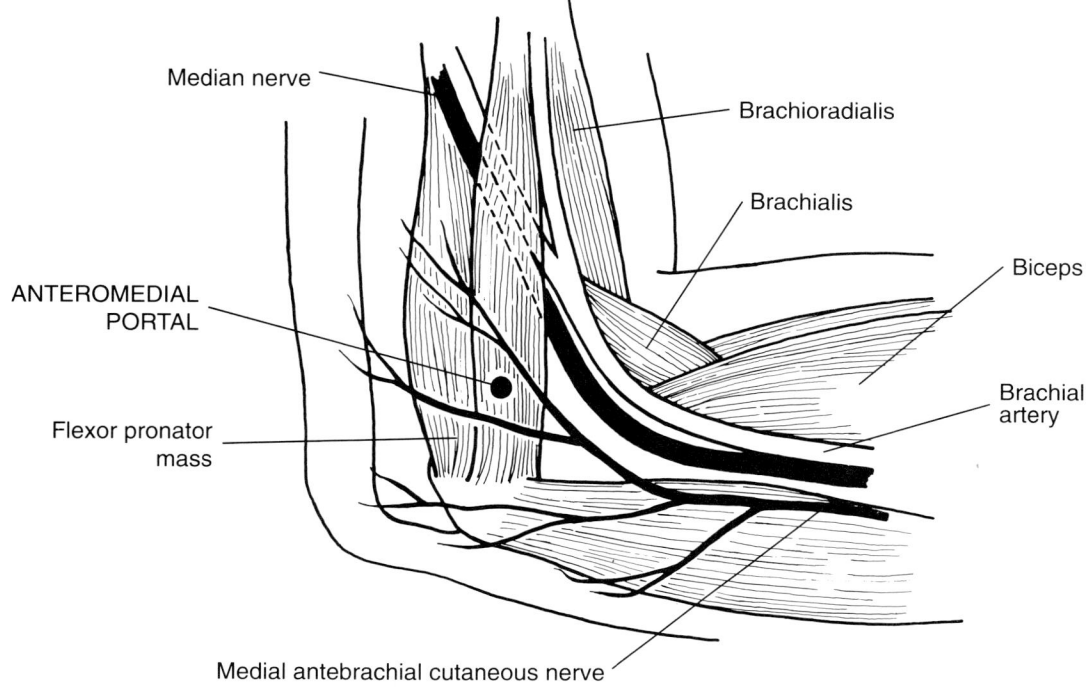

FIG 4–16. Anatomy of the medial antebrachial cutaneous nerve. (Modified from Lynch GJ, et al: *Arthroscopy* 2:192, 1986.)

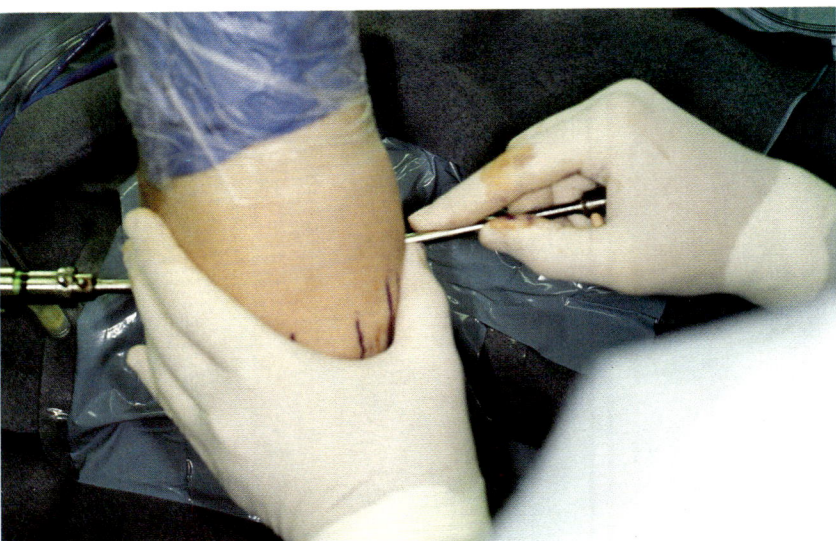

FIG 4–17. Example of blunt trocar being inserted through the anteromedial portal under direct visualization with the arthroscope in the anterolateral portal.

elbow is being maintained at all times, the extracapsular extravasation of the fluid should be monitored closely. Extracapsular extravasation is most often seen when repeated attempts have been made to establish the arthroscopic portals, resulting in multiple holes in the capsule and fluid leakage. When an inflow cannula is used as a separate portal for distention, the cannula should not have any "side vents," because if the inflow cannula slips back somewhat during the arthroscopic procedure, fluid will leak directly into the subcutaneous tissues.

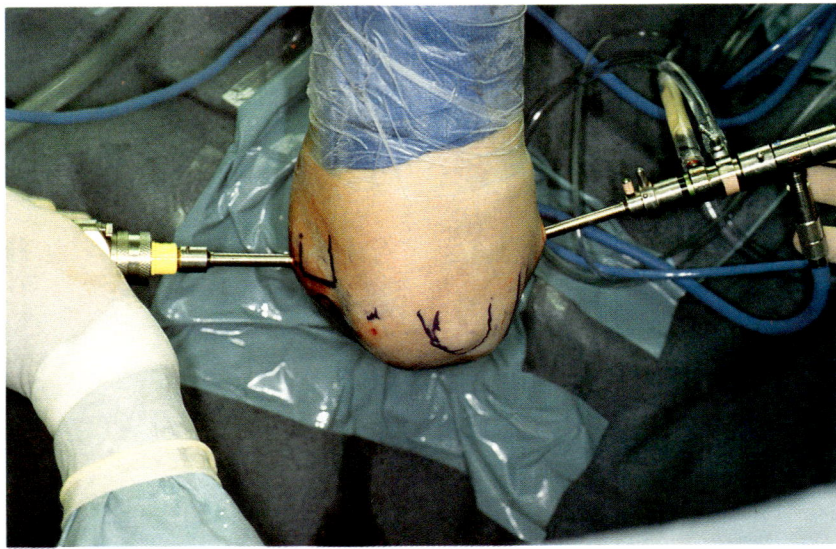

FIG 4–18. Example of arthroscope in place through the anteromedial portal, with a shaver in the anterolateral portal.

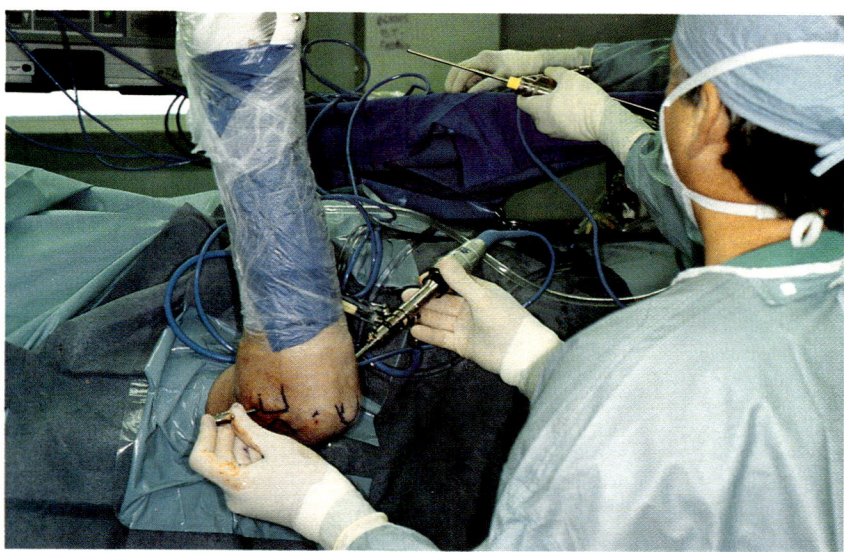

FIG 4–19. When the arthroscope is used in the anteromedial portal, it is helpful for the surgeon to sit at the medial aspect of the arm.

Most arthroscopic surgical procedures in the elbow are performed because of pathologic processes located over the lateral aspect of the elbow, such as loose bodies or osteochondritis dissecans of the capitellum. Therefore, one needs to be proficient in establishing both the anterolateral and the anteromedial portals. The anteromedial portal provides excellent visualization of the lateral aspect of the anterior compartment, compared with that provided through the actual anterolateral portal (Fig 4–18).

When the anterolateral portal is used for the arthroscope, the surgeon sits at the lateral or radial aspect of the arm. If the surgeon attempts to use the anteromedial portal for the arthroscope and still sits at the lateral or radial aspect of the arm, the arthroscope will be coming directly backward toward the surgeon, and orientation can be somewhat confusing when this is viewed on a video monitor. Therefore, if the surgeon is at the lateral aspect of the arm and using a medial arthroscopic portal, the surgeon should change position and sit at the medial aspect of the arm; this will greatly aid in orientation and maneuvering within the elbow joint (Fig 4–19).

As with establishment of the anterolateral arthroscopic portal, the elbow should be flexed 90 degrees at all times and maximum fluid distention should be maintained during establishment of the anteromedial arthroscopic portal. Lynch et al[24] demonstrated that with 35 to 40 mL fluid injected into the elbow, the median nerve and brachial artery are displaced anteriorly by 10 mm and 8 mm, respectively, from the entering arthroscopic instruments.

Direct Straight Lateral Portal

The direct lateral or soft spot portal is located in the triangular area bordered by the lateral humeral epicondyle, the radial head, and the olecranon (see Fig 4–5). Through this portal the trocar system passes through the anconeus muscle and the posterior capsule, the same area in which the 18-gauge spinal needle is inserted for initial distention of the elbow joint. This portal may be established without direct visualization by using an 18-

gauge spinal needle and the sharp and blunt trocar system. When this portal is established, the posterior antebrachial cutaneous nerve should be avoided.

When an arthroscopic pump is used, one may leave the 4-mm arthroscope in the anterolateral or anteromedial compartment to allow fluid inflow into the elbow joint. After the lateral portal is made with the knife, the small 2.7-mm arthroscope is placed through it (Fig 4–20). The small arthroscope is often advantageous in this small, tight area of the elbow joint. Cannulas have been adapted for the small arthroscope so that distention and pressure sensing are possible. Alternatively, one may use the 4-mm arthroscope.

Lateral Accessory Portal

An accessory lateral portal can be made at this point, if needed. The 18-gauge needle is inserted through the skin approximately 2 cm distal to the lateral portal. The needle is aimed toward the tip of the arthroscope. Once the needle is visualized, the portal is made with a knife, and a blunt trocar or shaver may be placed through it. This area of the elbow joint is usually a small space, and it is not uncommon to inadvertently pull the arthroscope or shaver out of the joint. Rotation of the arthroscope at 30 degrees rather than moving the arthroscope to change the view will help to prevent this. If the accessory lateral and lateral portals are made too close to each other, "crowding" will occur and triangulation will be awkward.

Posterolateral Portal

Arthroscopic evaluation of the elbow is not complete until the posterior structures have been visualized. The posterolateral portal is established approximately 3 cm proximal to the tip of the olecranon, just proximal and posterior to the lateral humeral epicondyle, along the lateral epicondylar ridge near the lateral border of the triceps muscle (Fig 4–

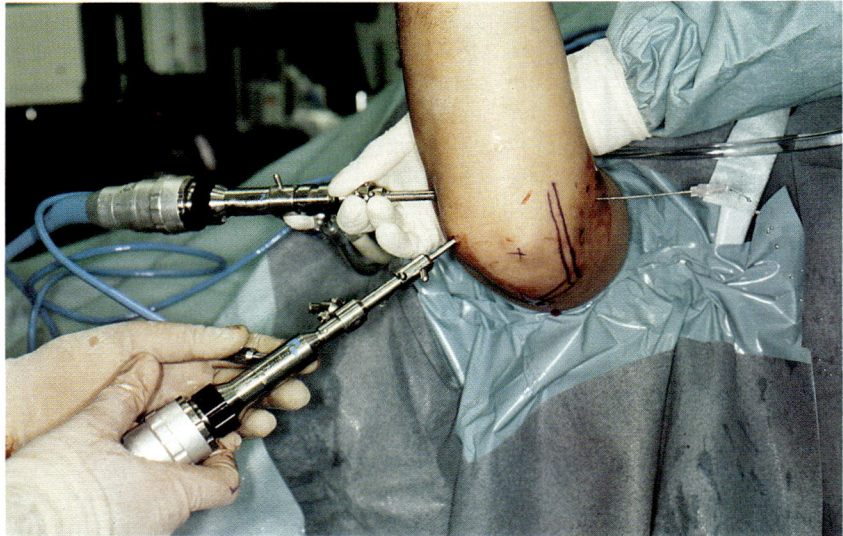

FIG 4–20. **A,** 4-mm arthroscope is in the anterolateral portal, and a 2.7-mm arthroscope in the direct lateral portal.

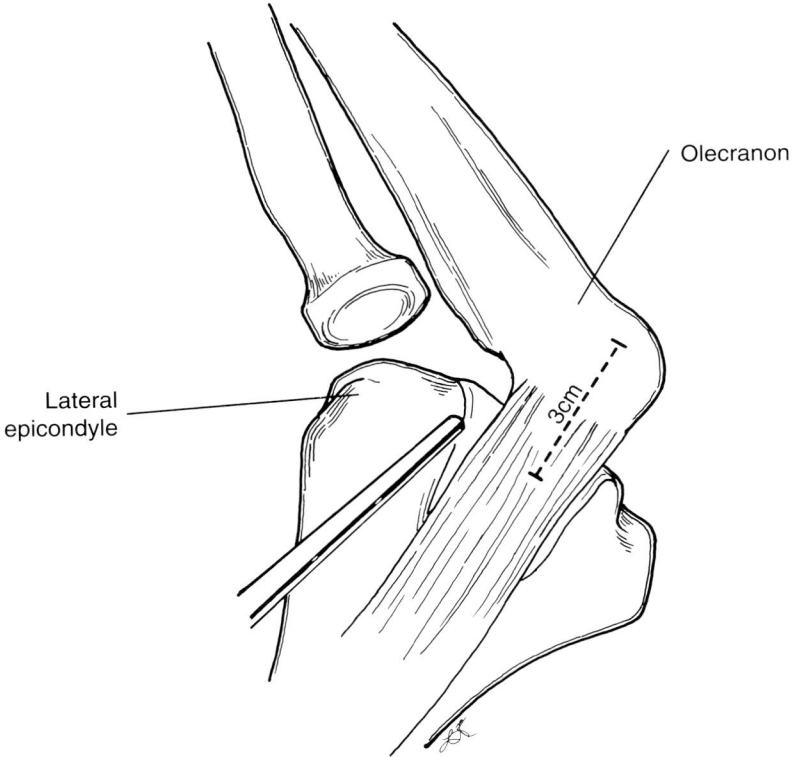

FIG 4–21. Posterolateral portal is located approximately 3 cm proximal to the olecranon tip, just superior and posterior to the lateral humeral epicondyle and off of the lateral border of the triceps muscle.

21). This portal is established with the elbow in 20 to 30 degrees of flexion under direct visualization. This extension of the elbow relaxes the posterior soft tissues and enlarges the space available for arthroscopy in the posterior compartment. With the arthroscope in the lateral portal, one follows the trochlear notch from distal to proximal until the posterolateral aspect of the olecranon tip is in view.[4] An 18-gauge spinal needle is placed through the previously marked posterolateral portal site and directed toward the olecranon fossa (Fig 4–22). After visualization of the needle, one incises the skin sharply with a knife. At times, some synovial tissue must be removed to allow visualization of the spinal needle. The arthroscopist may observe the knife entering into the joint, paralleling the spinal needle. The blunt trocar and sheath and then the arthroscope may be placed (Figs 4–22 to 4–24). The posterior antebrachial cutaneous nerve that courses over the posterolateral aspect of the distal humerus and the lateral brachial cutaneous nerve are to be avoided in establishment of this posterolateral portal (Fig 4–25).

Straight Posterior (Transtriceps) Portal

The straight posterior or transtriceps portal is located approximately 2 cm medial to the posterolateral portal and directly traverses the triceps tendon (Fig 4–26). The elbow is flexed 20 to 30 degrees. The portal is established by placing a spinal needle through the area under direct visualization. With the arthroscope in the posterolateral portal, the skin over the needle is incised in the direction of the triceps fibers (Fig 4–27). The straight

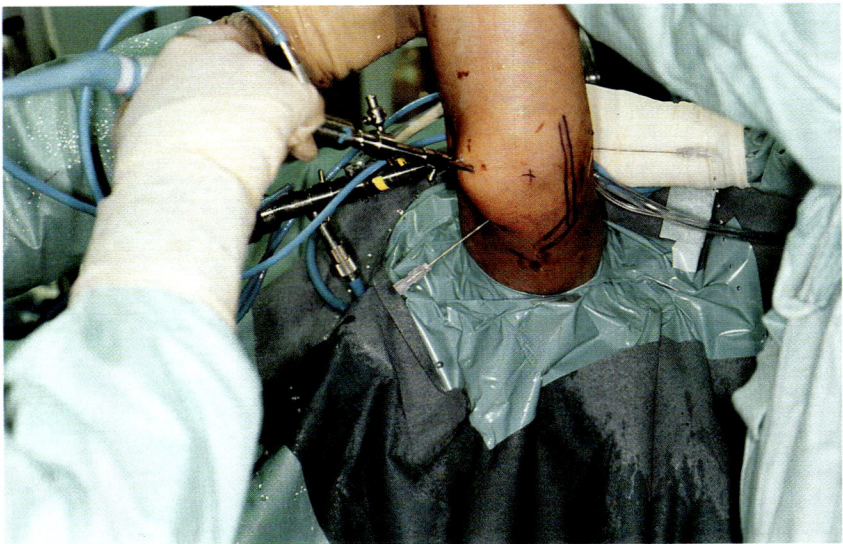

FIG 4–22. A 4-mm arthroscope is in the anterolateral portal, and a 2.7-mm arthroscope in the direct lateral portal, allowing visualization of the 18-gauge spinal needle placed through the posterolateral portal.

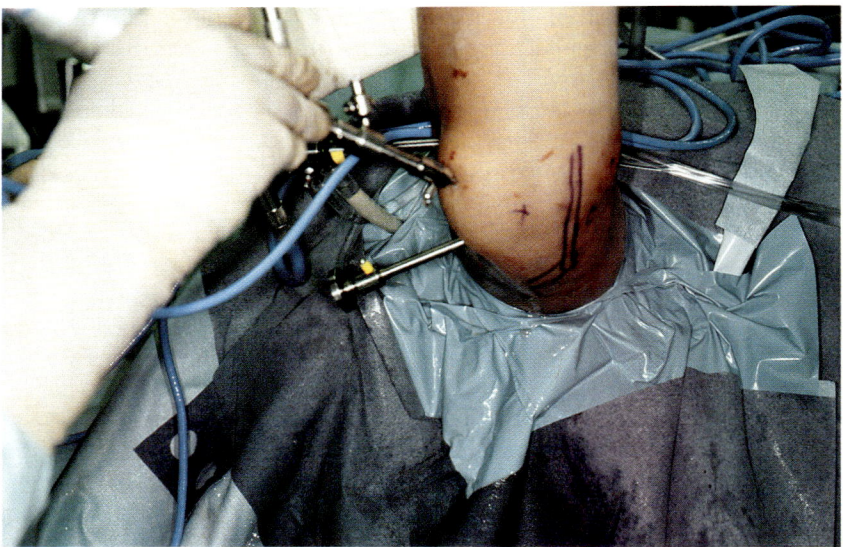

FIG 4–23. A 2.7-mm arthroscope in the direct lateral portal visualizes the blunt trocar placed through the posterolateral portal.

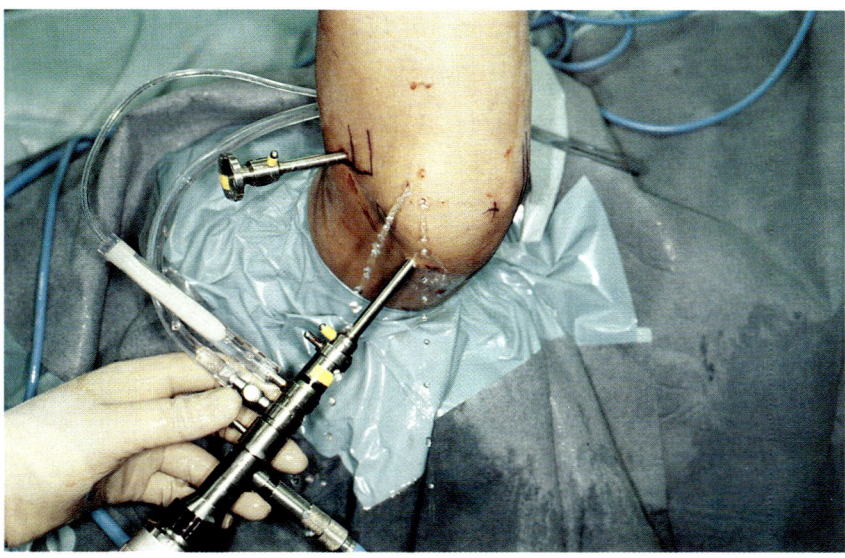

FIG 4–24. The 4-mm arthroscope is removed from the anterolateral portal and placed in the posterolateral portal. The 2.7-mm arthroscope is removed from the direct lateral portal.

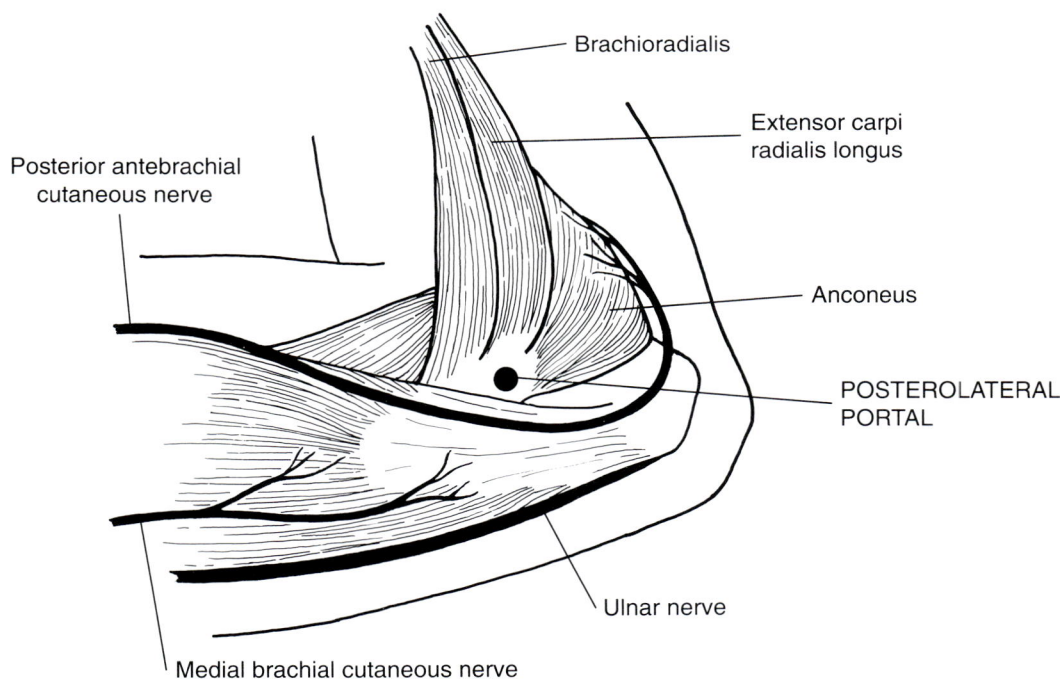

FIG 4–25. Anatomy of the posterior antebrachial cutaneous nerve. (Modified from Lynch GJ, et al: *Arthroscopy* 2:192, 1986.)

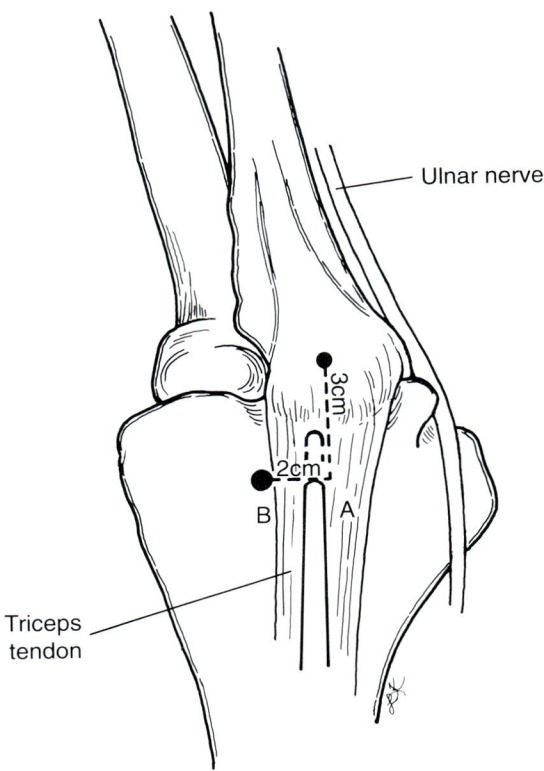

FIG 4–26. Straight posterior or transtriceps portal (**A**) is located 2 cm medial to the standard posterolateral portal (**B**) and passes directly through the triceps tendon.

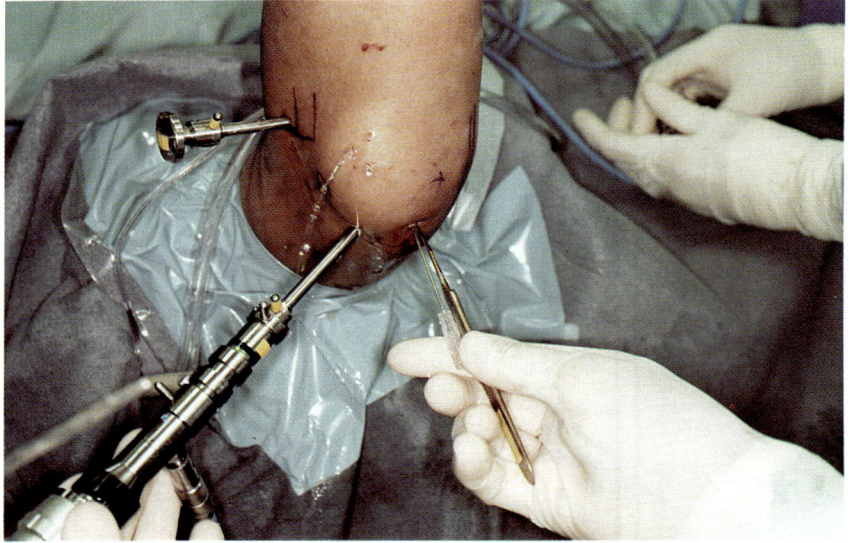

FIG 4–27. The 4-mm arthroscope is in the posterolateral portal. To establish the transtriceps portal, a knife is used to incise the skin over the 18-gauge needle.

posterior portal is the "working" portal posteriorly, and is useful for removing loose bodies from the posterior aspect of the elbow and the occasional resection of an impinging olecranon osteophyte.[3]

POEHLING SURGICAL TECHNIQUE

Some surgeons have proposed placing the patient in a prone position for elbow arthroscopy.[5, 17, 23, 29] This position provides ready access to both the anterior and posterior aspects of the elbow and allows gravity to help move the neurovascular structures in the antecubital fossa away from the entering instruments. Poehling et al[29] believe this position improves mobility because it does not require a traction suspension system. They assert that the prone position of the arm is more stable than the supine position with the arm suspended in an overhead traction apparatus. When used in conjunction with a proximal medial portal as the initial arthroscopic portal, the instruments enter more parallel to the neurovascular structures and possibly may protect these structures in initiation of the arthroscopic portal.[23] An improved view of the anterior joint with use of this portal has also been reported.[23]

When this technique is used, the patient is placed in the prone position (Fig 4–28) with the shoulder and proximal portion of the arm elevated on a sandbag, which is placed on an arm board adjacent to the operating table. The usual bony landmarks, including the medial and lateral humeral epicondyle, the medial intramuscular septum, the radial head, and the olecranon, are outlined with a marking pen. The joint is distended with

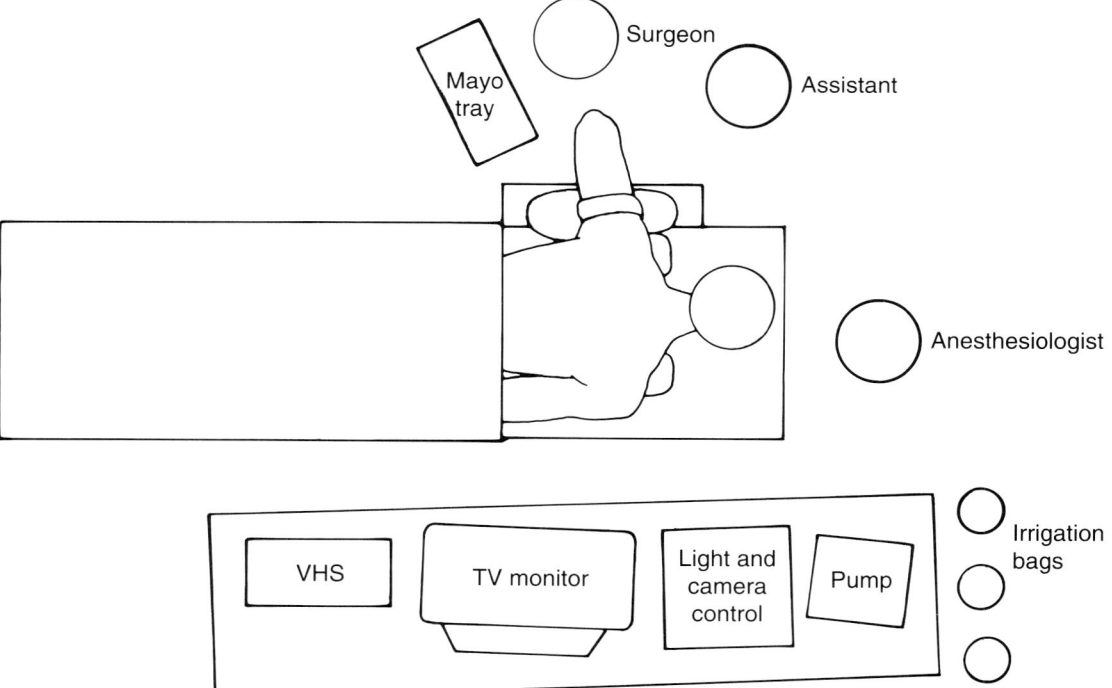

FIG 4–28. Operating room setup for arthroscopy of the left elbow with the patient in the prone position. (Modified from Poehling GG et al: *Arthroscopy* 5:222, 1989.)

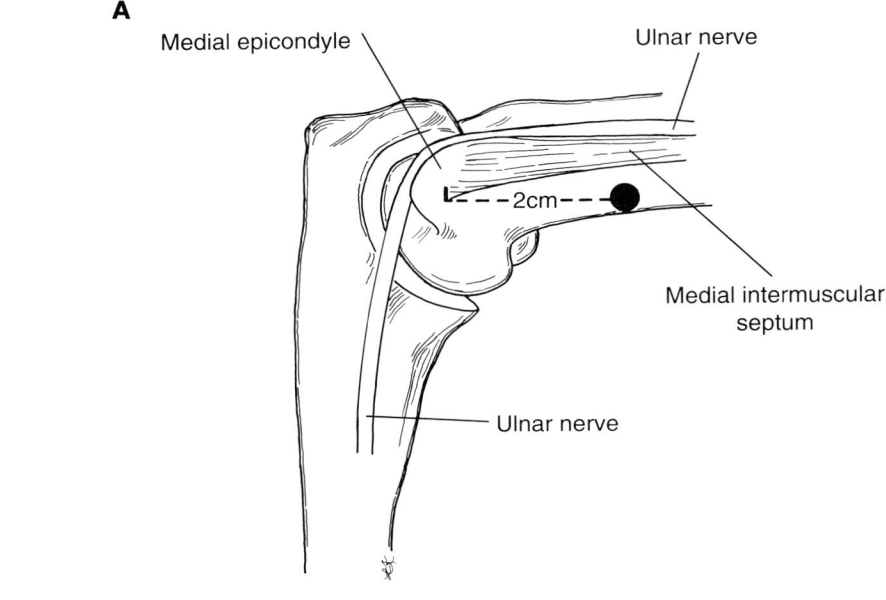
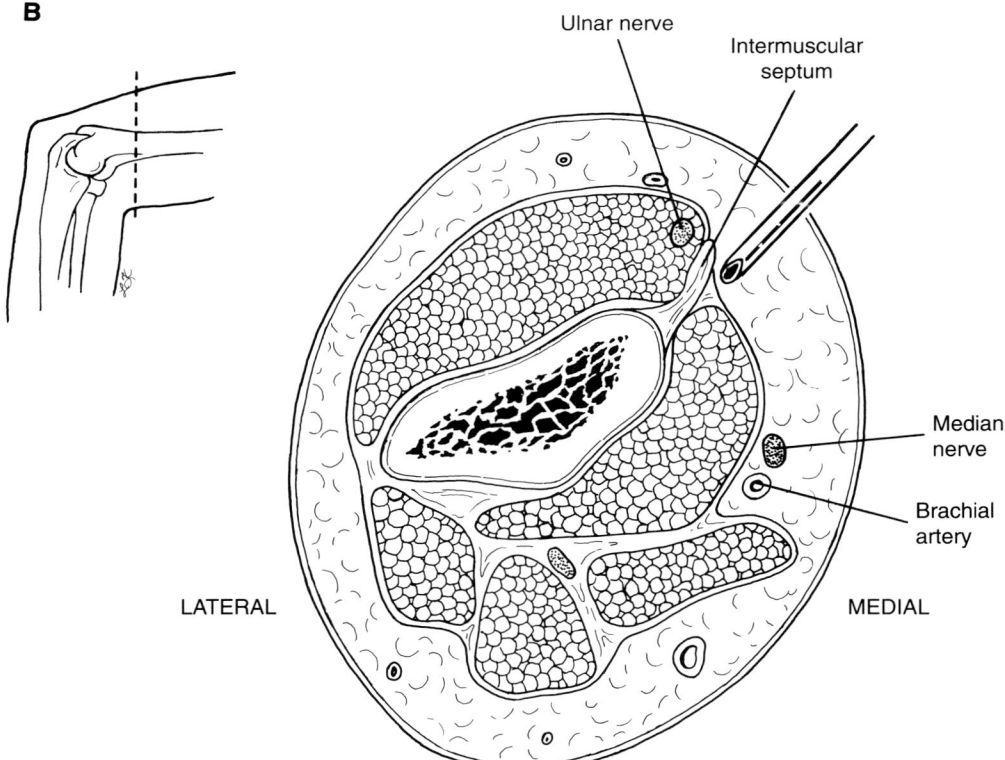

FIG 4–29. **A,** insertion site for the proximal medial portal is located 2 cm proximal to the medial humeral epicondyle and anterior to the palpable medial intermuscular septum. **B,** cross-sectional view of the proximal medial portal. Sheath and blunt trocar are inserted anterior to the intermuscular septum and in contact with the anterior humerus, which is directed toward the radial head to avoid injury to the neurovascular structures. (Modified from Poehling GG, et al: *Arthroscopy* 5:222, 1989.)

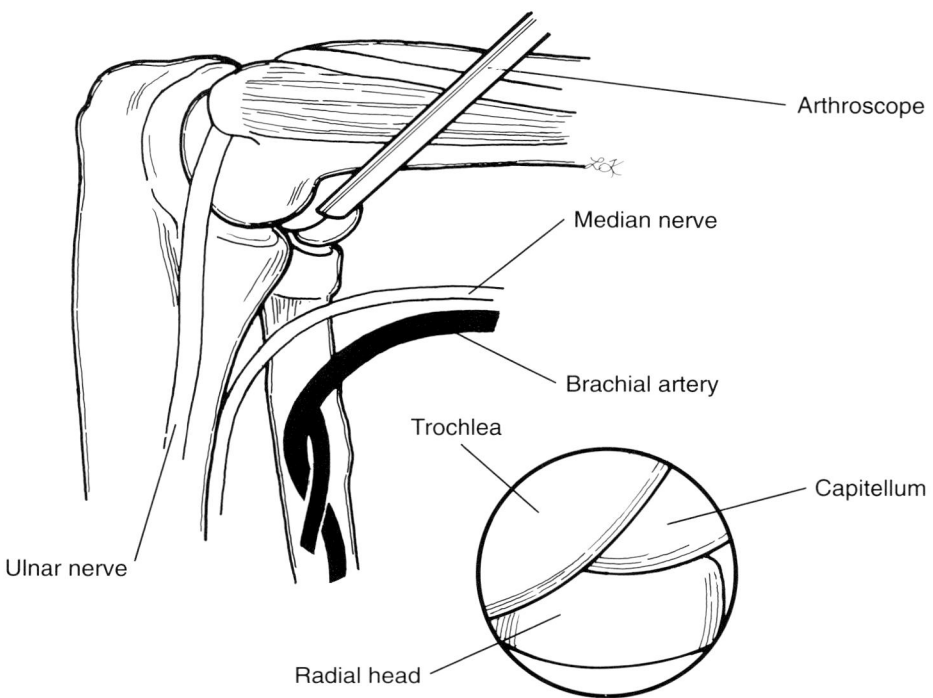

FIG 4–30. Arthroscopic view of anterior aspect of the elbow, obtained by using the proximal medial portal. (Modified from Poehling GG, et al: *Arthroscopy* 5:222, 1989.)

30 to 40 mL of fluid injected into the elbow laterally through the soft spot bordered by the radial head, olecranon, and lateral humeral epicondyle. The proximal medial portal is located 2 cm proximal to the medial humeral epicondyle (Fig 4–29,A). Injury to the ulnar nerve may be avoided by remaining anterior to the easily palpated intramuscular septum. A small skin incision is made with the tip of a No. 11 scalpel blade. The cannula and blunt trocar are then inserted, anterior to the intramuscular septum and in contact with the anterior humerus (Fig 4–29,B). The trocar is directed toward the radial head during insertion. The elbow capsule is then punctured, and the arthroscope is inserted. Because the arthroscope is entering more proximal than in the anteromedial or anterolateral portals, the overall view of the anterior aspect of the elbow is increased (Fig 4–30).

Cadaveric dissection studies[23,24,34] have demonstrated that there is increased distance between the instruments and the neurovascular structures when the proximal medial arthroscopic portal is used as the initial diagnostic portal, compared with when the anterolateral portal is used, with which there is less distance between the instruments and the radial nerve (see Chapter 7).

POSTOPERATIVE ROUTINE

At the completion of the arthroscopic procedure, thorough irrigation of the joint can greatly improve the postoperative recovery. Irrigation is particularly important in debridement of adhesions or of articular surfaces. This step is often neglected because of the belief that the joint has been sufficiently irrigated during the operative procedure. The elbow cannot be flexed and extended completely with all the instruments in place, however, and larger material can be removed from an open cannula system than from one that has an arthroscope in place. Thus, at the end of the surgical procedure, one inflow cannula is left in place, the elbow is completely flexed and extended several times, and irrigation and suction are alternated to remove any debris. The arthroscopic portals may be closed with suture material or left open, depending on the preference of the surgeon and the amount of subcutaneous swelling. We usually leave portals open. We do not recommend the use of local anesthetics for postoperative pain control, because they may leak out of the capsular holes and cause a temporary nerve block,[1,26] which would interfere with the immediate postoperative neurovascular assessment. A drain may be placed through the anterior and/or posterior portals if extensive debridement has been performed. Soft dressings are applied to the elbow, and in most cases immobilization is not required. Active range of motion of the elbow is initiated as soon as pain and swelling permit. Strengthening exercises are initiated when sufficient range of motion has been achieved and when pain and swelling permit. See the discussion on postoperative rehabilitation in Chapter 8.

SUMMARY

Arthroscopy of the elbow is a technically demanding surgical procedure, and careful attention to detail is essential to perform a safe and reproducible arthroscopic examinaton. It is important that the skin be properly marked before initiation of the surgical procedure, to maintain proper orientation at all times. Also, the use of an 18-gauge spinal needle as a precursor to the larger arthroscopic instruments is recommended. The elbow should be kept flexed at 90 degrees, and maximally distended with fluids to relax the neurovascular structures and to move these structures away from the arthroscopic instruments except when working in the posterior compartment where less flexion is desired. One must constantly palpate the anterior portion of the elbow during the procedure, to detect extravasation of fluid and compression of the neurovascular bundle. Complications may be avoided by adhering to a strict surgical technique.

REFERENCES

1. Andrews JR, Carson WG: Arthroscopy of the elbow, *Arthroscopy* 1:97–107, 1985.
2. Andrews JR, Carson WG: Arthroscopy of the elbow. In McGinty JB, editor: *Techniques in orthopaedics: arthroscopic surgery update,* Rockville, Md, 1985 Aspen Systems, pp 183–190.
3. Andrews JR, St. Pierre RK, Carson WG: Arthroscopy of the elbow, *Clin Sports Med* 5:653–662, 1986.
4. Andrews JR, Craven WM: Lesions of the posterior compartment of the elbow, *Clin Sports Med* 10:637–652, 1991.
5. Baker CL, Shalvoy RM: The prone position for elbow arthroscopy, *Clin Sports Med* 10:623–628, 1991.
6. Boe S: Arthroscopy of the elbow: diagnosis and extraction of loose bodies, *Acta Orthop Scand* 57:52–53, 1986.
7. Burman MS: Arthroscopy or the direct visualization of joints, *J Bone Joint Surg* 13:669–695, 1931.
8. Carson WG: Arthroscopy of the elbow. In Zarins B, Andrews J, Carson WG, editors: *Injuries to the throwing arm,* Philadelphia, 1985, WB Saunders, pp 221–227.
9. Carson WG: Arthroscopy of the elbow. *Instr Course Lect* 37:195–201, 1988.
10. Carson WG: Complications of elbow arthroscopy. In Minkoff J, Sherman O, editors: *Arthroscopic surgery,* Baltimore, 1988, Williams & Wilkins, pp 166–179.

11. Carson WG: Arthroscopy of the elbow. In Torg J, Welsh RP, editors: *Current therapy in sports medicine*, Philadelphia, 1988, BC Decker.
12. Carson WG, Meyers JF: Diagnostic arthroscopy of the elbow: surgical technique and arthroscopic portal anatomy. In McGinty JB, editor: *Operative arthroscopy*, New York, 1991, Raven Press, pp 583–594.
13. Casscells SW: Neurovascular anatomy and elbow arthroscopy: inherent risks (editor's comment), *Arthroscopy* 2:190, 1987.
14. DeLee JC: Complications of arthroscopy and arthroscopic surgery: results of a national survey, *Arthroscopy* 1:214–220, 1985.
15. Eriksson E, Denti M: Diagnostic and operative arthroscopy of the shoulder and elbow joint, *Ital J Sports Traumatol* 7:165–188, 1985.
16. Guhl JF: Arthroscopy and arthroscopic surgery of the elbow, *Orthopedics* 8:290–296, 1985.
17. Hempfling H: Die endoskopisch Untersuching des Ellenbogen-gelenkes vom dorso-radialen Zugang, *Z Orthop* 121:331, 1983.
18. Ito K: The arthroscopic anatomy of the elbow joint, *Arthroscopy* 4:2–9, 1979 (Japanese literature).
19. Ito K: Arthroscopy of the elbow joint: a cadaver study, *Arthroscopy* 5:9–22, 1980 (Japanese literature).
20. Ito K: Arthroscopy of the elbow joint, *Arthroscopy* 6:15–24, 1981.
21. Ito K: Arthroscopy of the elbow joint. In Watanabe M, editor: *Arthroscopy of small joints*, New York, 1985, Igaku-Shoin, pp 57–84.
22. Johnson LL: Elbow arthroscopy. In *Arthroscopic surgery: principles and practice*, St Louis, 1986, Mosby, pp 1446–1477.
23. Lindenfeld TN: Medial approach to elbow arthroscopy, *Am J Sports Med* 18:413–417, 1990.
24. Lynch GJ, et al: Neurovascular anatomy and elbow arthroscopy: inherent risks, *Arthroscopy* 2:191–197, 1986.
25. Maeda Y: Arthroscopy of the elbow joint, *Arthroscopy* 5:5–8, 1980 (Japanese literature).
26. Morrey BF: Arthroscopy of the elbow, *Instr Course Lect* 35:102, 1986.
27. O'Driscoll SW, Morrey BF, Au KN: Intraarticular pressure and capacity of the elbow, *Arthroscopy* 6:100–103, 1990.
28. Papilion JD, Neff RS, Shall LM: Compression neuropathy of the radial nerve as a complication of elbow arthroscopy: a case report and review of the literature, *Arthroscopy* 4:284–286, 1988.
29. Poehling GG, et al: Elbow arthroscopy: a new technique, *Arthroscopy* 5:222–224, 1989.
30. Ruch DS, Poehling GG: Arthroscopic treatment of Panner's disease, *Clin Sports Med* 10:629–636, 1991.
31. Schonholtz GJ: *Arthroscopic surgery of the shoulder, elbow and ankle*, Springfield, Ill, 1986, Charles C Thomas, pp 73–78.
32. Small NC: Complications in arthroscopy: on knee and other joints, *Arthroscopy* 2:253–258, 1986.
33. Thomas MA, Fast A, Shapiro D: Radial nerve damage as a complication of elbow arthroscopy, *Clin Orthop* 214:130–131, 1987.
34. Verhaar J, VanMameren H, Brandsma A: Risks of neurovascular injury in elbow arthroscopy: starting anteromedially or anterolaterally?, *Arthroscopy* 7:287–290, 1991.
35. Watanabe M: Arthroscopy of small joints, *J Jpn Orthop Assoc* 45:908, 1971 (Japanese literature).
36. Woods GW: Elbow arthroscopy, *Clin Sports Med* 6:557, 1987.

Chapter 5

Arthroscopic Surgical Procedures of the Elbow: Common Cases

Stephen R. Soffer, M.D.
James R. Andrews, M.D.

LOOSE BODY REMOVAL

Loose bodies in the elbow may be secondary to joint surface disintegration (e.g., degenerative joint disease or osteochondritis dissecans), proliferative diseases of the synovium (e.g., synovial chondromatosis), or osteochondral fractures.[2, 17] The most common cause is probably joint surface fragmentation.[17] Regardless of their origin, once these bodies become loose a common sequence of morphologic alterations occurs. This process, well described by Milgram[17] in 1977, involves proliferation of bone and cartilage as well as osteoclastic resorption on the surfaces of these free bodies. Chondroblasts, osteoblasts, and osteoclasts receive nutrition from synovial fluid and proliferate. Bone and cartilage then forms on loose body surfaces. As loose bodies grow in size, diffusion of synovial fluid nutrients to deeper layers becomes minimal and cellular necrosis with secondary dystrophic calcification ensues. Osteoclastic resorption creates the pitting on loose body surfaces.

A typical case usually involves a male athlete, often a weight lifter or football player, aged 25 to 45 years. The patient complains of loss of motion, especially extension,[1] and may also complain of catching, locking, or grating. Routine radiographs, including anteroposterior, lateral, oblique, and axial views, may show opaque densities or degenerative joint disease. Radiographs often are negative, especially if the loose bodies are cartilaginous and noncalcified. Even computed tomography (CT) scans and magnetic resonance (MR) images may not allow identification of these entities. In these situations, arthroscopy is helpful in diagnosis and treatment of loose bodies in the elbow.

Before arthroscopy for loose body removal, it is prudent to inform the patient and his or her family of three important concepts:

1. The loose body may not be found at the time of surgery.
2. There may be more than one loose body in the joint.
3. Loose bodies can "recur." More accurately, not all loose bodies may be seen at the initial surgery; therefore, the patient may need additional surgery in the fu-

ture for loose body removal. Another possibility is that the primary disease process (e.g., degenerative joint disease, chondromatosis) is not cured and may continue to produce loose bodies.

Preoperative discussion of these three ideas is extremely important to prevent ill feelings, misunderstandings, and disappointment between patient and doctor.

Technique

Finding Loose Bodies. To locate loose bodies arthroscopically can at times be difficult and frustrating. The primary pathologic condition (e.g., osteoarthritis, osteochondritis dissecans, synovial chondromatosis) is a helpful clue as to loose body location. For example, loose bodies associated with an arthritic elbow will often be near the tips of the olecranon and coronoid. Laterally located loose bodies are often seen with osteochondritis dissecans of the capitellum or radial head. In proliferate diseases of the synovium (e.g., synovial chondromatosis) most loose bodies will be in the anterior compartment adherent to the synovium. Loose bodies caused by fractures are usually near the coronoid, olecranon tip, and radial head. Surgery for each of these disease processes is discussed in other chapters.

Even the best arthroscopist may have difficulty finding a loose body despite a thorough, diagnostic arthroscopy of all compartments and gutters. Placing a shaver in each compartment, with full suction, may help to bring forth these loose bodies. One must be cartain to investigate the dependent, posterior compartment and the lateral gutter, where loose bodies often reside. In fact, loose bodies visualized in the anterior compartment during arthroscopy often migrate to these areas because of the inflow pressure gradient and gravity dependence.

Multiple Loose Bodies. After a loose body seen on preoperative radiographs has been found, the operation is not over. The arthroscopist should perform a thorough and complete diagnostic arthroscopic examination. One will often find additional pathologic processes or additional loose bodies in the other compartments of the elbow. For example, in an arthritic elbow, it is not uncommon to find a loose body in the anterior compartment, associated with the coronoid, along with an osteophyte or loose body in the posterior compartment, associated with the olecranon tip or olecranon fossa.

In the case of multiple loose bodies in the anterior compartment, establishment of the anteromedial portal may be difficult because the anteromedial aspect of the anterior compartment is obscured by loose bodies. Also, visualization of the localizing 18-gauge needle placed anteromedially may be difficult because of multiple loose bodies. In this situation one must keep the arthroscope in a position to give a wide view of the medial side. A common mistake is to place the arthroscope too far into the joint, close to the obscuring loose bodies, which produces a crowding effect. In this position, it will be difficult to find the localizing needle, because the field of view is limited by the loose bodies. With the arthroscope in the anterolateral portal and a more panoramic view of the anterior compartment, the needle is placed medially through the previously marked medial portal entry point (2 cm distal and 2 cm anterior to the medial epicondyle).

Palpation of the humerus with the needle may be attempted. The surgeon places the needle directly onto the distal humerus, through the previously marked anteromedial portal. By moving the needle anteriorly while palpating the distal humerus, the needle will then "fall into" the anterior compartment. Then, while looking anteromedially from the anterolateral compartment, one "wiggles" the needle. By moving the arthroscope toward this motion, the needle can usually be found.

Another technique to establish an anteromedial portal may prove helpful. With the arthroscope in the anterolateral portal, the arthroscope is directed anteromedially toward the humeroulnar articulation. The operating room overhead lights are dimmed, and the light from the arthroscope can be seen shining through the skin, anteromedially. One may also palpate the tip of the arthroscope against the skin, just anterior and distal to the medial epicondyle. An 18-gauge needle is placed directly on this point, and the arthroscope is retracted (i.e., pulled anterolaterally approximately 1 inch) as the needle is advanced into the joint.

The "Wissinger rod" technique may also be useful in establishment of the anteromedial portal. As described in the preceding paragraph, the arthroscope is placed against the anteromedial joint capsule just proximal and anterior to the ulnohumeral articulation. The arthroscope is removed from the cannula. A Wissinger rod is placed through the cannula and is pressed against the anteromedial capsule and skin. With a No. 11 blade, the surgeon incises the skin over the rod, which is easily palpated anteromedially. The rod is passed through the skin. Then, a cannula is placed over the end of the rod and the anteromedial cannula introduced into the joint. Once the anteromedial cannula is in the joint, the Wissinger rod is removed and the arthroscope is placed back into the anterolateral portal. The large-bore anteromedial cannula should be easily visualized.

Now that both portals in the anterior compartment have been established, one places the arthroscope in first the anterolateral portal, then the anteromedial portal, to verify that both portals are in the ideal position for efficient anterior compartment arthroscopic surgery. Small changes in portal location can be accomplished now by repuncturing the capsule under direct visualization. This will allow perfect positioning of both portals so that maximum benefit can be achieved from them. (One may need to remove some of the loose bodies, before this process, to aid in visualization.) In removal of loose bodies, use of a shaver rather than a loose body retriever prevents the risk of losing the established medial portal. After removal of all loose bodies in this fashion, the arthroscopist switches the arthroscope from the anterolateral to the anteromedial portal so that the entire anterior compartment may be visualized. More loose bodies can be removed by placing the shaver in the anterolateral portal.

In the knee, some arthroscopists recommend complete diagnostic arthroscopy of all compartments before any arthroscopic surgery (e.g., debridement, meniscectomy). However, in the elbow, it is usually wise to complete the diagnostic and arthroscopic surgery in each compartment as it is entered, rather than to perform initial diagnostic arthroscopy of the whole elbow joint (all three compartments). The former is a more organized, efficient, and safer method of elbow arthroscopy.

"Recurrence." Loose bodies are not always readily seen at the first arthroscopy. This is probably the most common reason for recurrence. The ongoing process of the primary pathologic condition, such as degenerative arthrosis and synovial chondromatosis, is the next most common reason. It is not a failure or complication of the first arthroscopy to need to remove more loose bodies by means of a second arthroscopy. This concept should be explained in detail to the patient before the initial surgery and should be reinforced afterward.

Case History

A 16-year-old high-school pitcher with a 2- to 3-year history of elbow pain complains of experiencing locking and clicking for 3 months (Figs 5–1-5–7.)

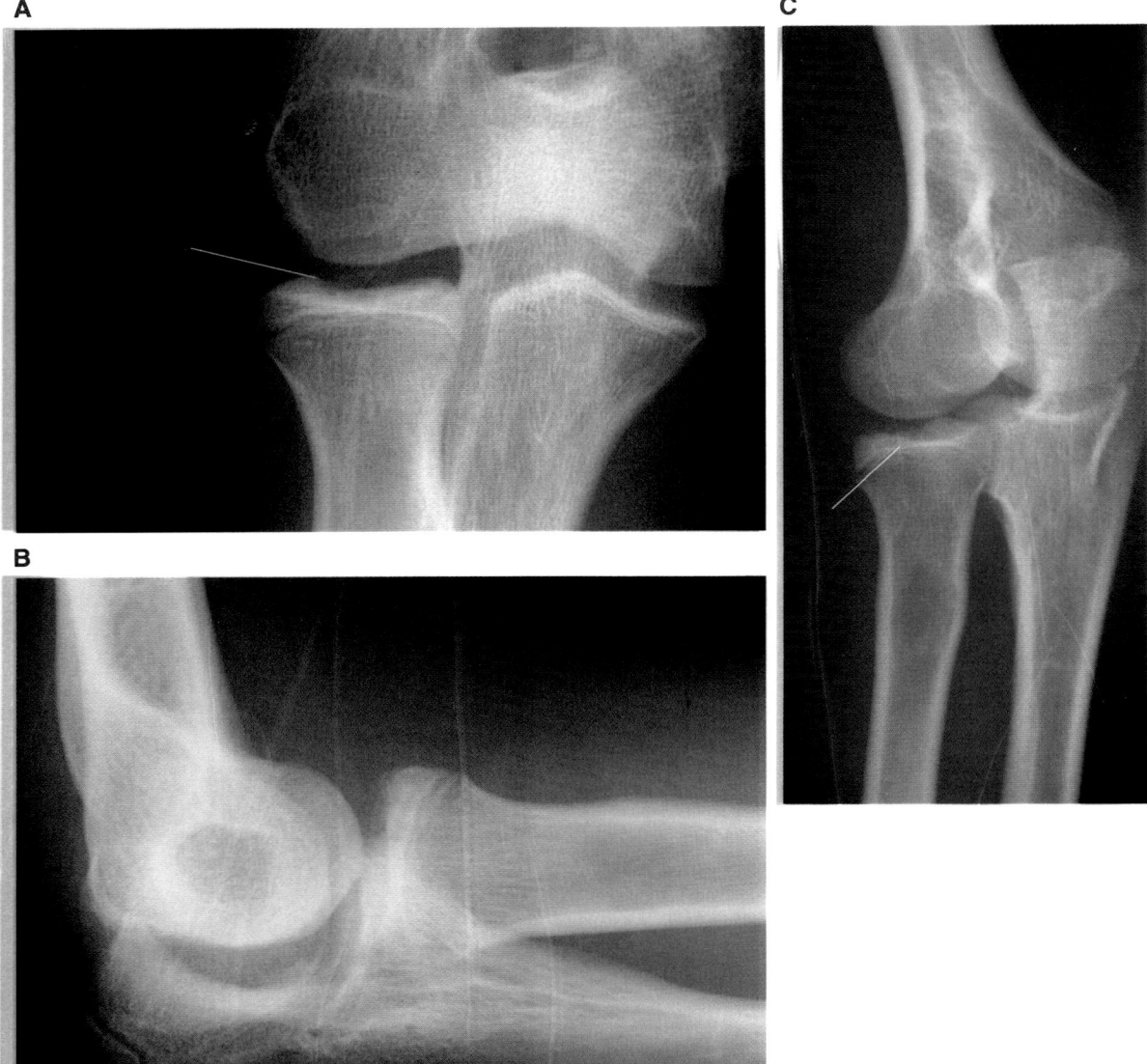

FIG 5–1. Anteroposterior (**A**), lateral (**B**), and oblique (**C**) radiographs reveal osteochondritis dissecans of the radial head with a loose body in the radiocapitellar compartment.

CHONDROPLASTY FOR OSTEOCHONDRITIS DISSECANS

The term osteochondritis dissecans was coined by Franz Konig more than 100 years ago.[13] Much confusion with regard to the terminology used in discussion of this disease exists because the disease is not fully understood. Panner's disease (or osteochondrosis of the capitellum) and osteochondritis dissecans are probably not two separate disease processes but different stages of the same progressive alteration of enchondral ossification.[25, 27]

The cause of this entity is controversial[6, 20, 23, 24, 33]; however, we agree with Singer and Roy[27] that osteochondritis dissecans of the capitellum is caused by repetitive micro-

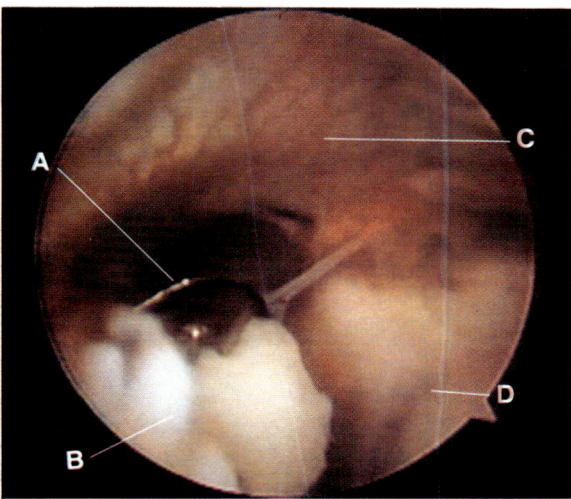

FIG 5-2. Loose bodies were found in the anterior compartment. An arthroscope is in the anterolateral portal. A loose body retriever *(a)* is in the anteromedial portal, poised to grasp the loose body *(b)*. *c*, medial capsule; *d*, anterior humerus.

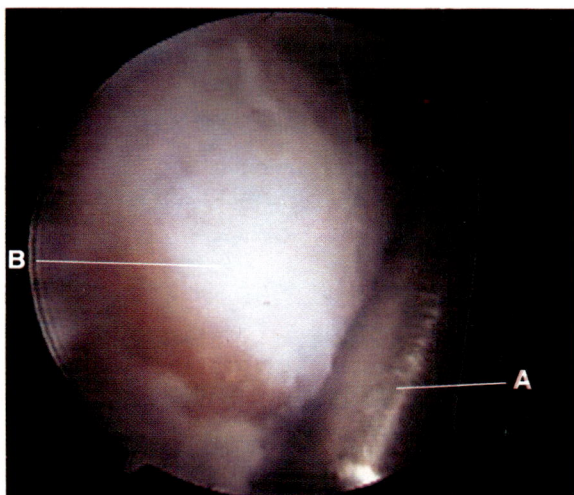

FIG 5-3. A second loose body is evident in the anterior compartment, adherent to the adjacent radiocapitellar joint. A shaver *(a)* debrides adhesions around the loose body to free up the loose body *(b)*.

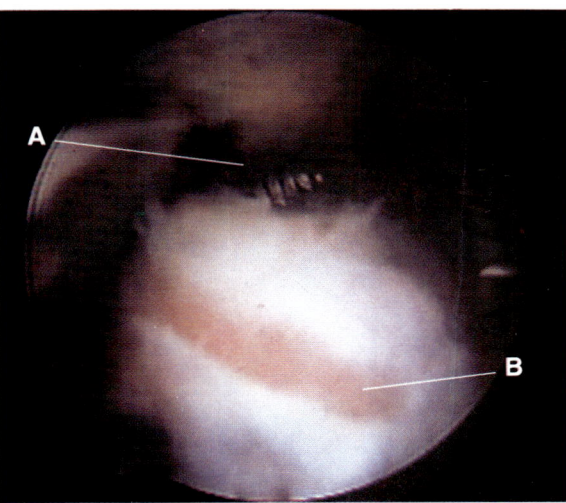

FIG 5-4. A loose body retriever *(a)* is used to remove the loose body *(b)*.

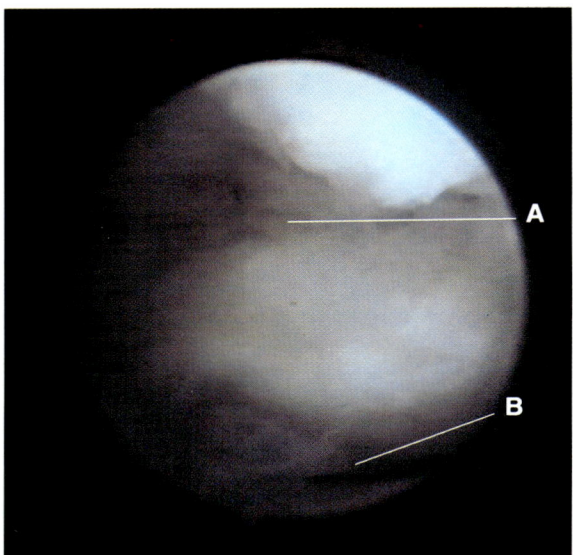

FIG 5–5. With the arthroscope in the lateral portal, an osteochondritic lesion of the radial head *(a)* is visualized. *b,* capitellum.

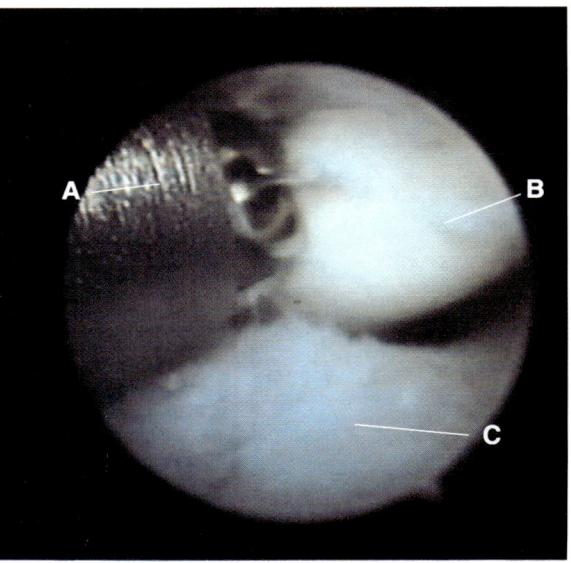

FIG 5–6. Through an accessory lateral portal, a shaver *(a)* is used to debride loose cartilage from the radial head lesion *(b)*. *c,* capitellum.

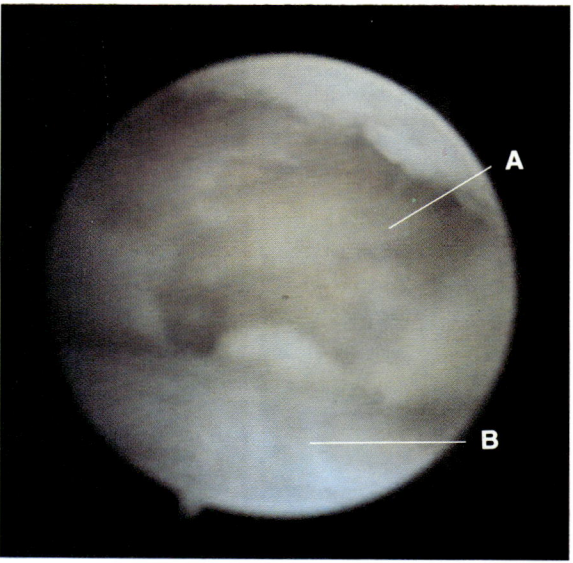

FIG 5–7. Radial head *(a)* after abrasion arthroplasty. Debridement of loose cartilage down to bleeding bone was performed. *b,* capitellum.

trauma to a vulnerable epiphysis with tenuous vascular supply. This is precipitated by compressive forces generated as a secondary component of medial valgus stress during athletic activity, such as throwing.[14, 29] Other possible causes include cartilage rests, bacterial embolism, fracture, hereditary abnormalities, and constitutional factors, among others.

Evaluation of pathologic specimens obtained from patients with osteochondritis dissecans in the knee revealed focal areas of avascular necrosis and repair of the subchondral bone of the epiphysis with normal appearing articular cartilage.[5]

The vascular anatomy of the distal humerus was extensively studied by Haraldsson.[9] He found that in the skeletally immature elbow, the capitellum's vascular supply consisted of just a few small vessels entering posteriorly. No vessels crossed the physis from the metaphysis. After physeal closure, vessels from the metaphysis crossed the physeal scar, and there were multiple anastomoses between the blood supplies of the epiphysis and metaphysis, causing the capitellum to be well vascularized. Thus, the blood supply to the capitellum is vulnerable in the skeletally immature.

A typical case usually involves a male thrower, aged 13 to 16 years, with complaints of dull pain on the lateral aspect of the elbow and loss of motion. He may complain of loose body–type symptoms, such as locking or catching. Examination will reveal decreased range of motion, especially extension, tenderness over the radiocapitellar joint, and often palpable crepitus.

Radiographs often, but not always, show irregularity of the capitellar surface or radiolucency of the capitellum. Tomograms, CT scans with contrast medium, or MR images are often helpful in establishment of the diagnosis.

Lesions are classified as intact (in situ), partially detached, or completely detached (loose body) (see Fig 5–1.) The detached portion may be cartilaginous or osteocartilaginous. Some authors base their treatment protocols on this classification.[21, 24] Drilling, internal fixation, bone grafting, debridement, or abrasion arthroplasty have been recommended after failure of conservative treatment.

Our indications for surgery for osteochondritis dissecans are failure of conservative treatment, loose bodies, and locked elbow. We have found that simple excision of loose or detached cartilage along with either chondroplasty or abrasion arthroplasty of the capitellum yields more gratifying results with quicker return to athletic activities than achieved with more complex procedures. Other authors agree.[16, 33]

Technique

Chondroplasty (i.e., debridement of articular cartilage) with arthroscopic guidance is commonly used as treatment for osteochondritic lesions of the radiocapitellar articulation. Although the technique that we will describe may be used for any cartilage debridement performed in the elbow, regardless of the cause, we will focus on chondroplasty for osteochondritis dissecans.

It is critical that thorough diagnostic arthroscopy be performed in a patient with osteochondritis dissecans. Other diagnoses should be ruled out, and all compartments should be inspected for loose bodies (see the preceeding section on loose bodies).

The arthroscopist establishes anterolateral and anteromedial portals as previously described. With the arthroscope in the anteromedial portal and a shaver in the anterolateral portal, the anterolateral aspect of the radiocapitellar joint can be visualized. The surgical assistant may flex and extend the elbow, pronate and supinate the forearm, and apply a varus stress (to open the radiocapitellar joint) to maximize visualization of this articulation. Loose cartilage should be debrided when encountered, and the radial notch and radial gutter should be inspected for loose fragments.

After anterior compartment surgery is completed, one proceeds to the lateral compartment. The area of osteochondritis is best seen with the arthroscope in the straight lateral portal. With the arthroscope in the lateral portal and a shaver in the accessory lateral portal, debriding of the often present synovitis that impedes full visualization of the lateral compartment is helpful. One then probes the osteochondritic lesion and determines its boundaries. With a shaver, banana blade, or basket forceps, the loose cartilage is excised. Usually, a shaver works best. Frequent rotation of an arthroscope angled at 30 degrees, rather than movement of the arthroscope, allows different perspectives of the elbow joint. This will avoid accidental withdrawal of the arthroscope from the elbow. The lateral compartment is a tight space, and minimal movements are necessary to prevent this occurrence.

At this point, one may switch portals, placing the arthroscope in the accessory lateral portal and the shaver in the lateral portal, for different view of the radiocapitellar joint. The forearm is rotated and the elbow is flexed and extended to complete evaluation of the entire radial head and capitellum. For example, flexing of the elbow to beyond 90 degrees is effective in uncovering capitellar lesions. The surgeon may use a Kirschner wire to drill or a burr to abrade the capitellum down to bleeding bone (see the following section on abrasion arthroplasty).

The arthroscopic examination for osteochondritis dissecans is complete after the posterior compartment has been evaluated in standard fashion. The surgeon should be certain to rule out loose bodies, posterior impingement, and additional diagnoses.

Case History

A 27-year-old professional baseball pitcher complains of right elbow pain over the radio capitellar compartment (Figs 5–8-5–12).

ABRASION ARTHROPLASTY FOR DEGENERATIVE JOINT DISEASE AND VALGUS EXTENSION OVERLOAD

Degenerative Joint Disease

Primary degenerative joint disease or osteoarthritis of the elbow is rare. The cause of degenerative joint disease of the elbow is multifaceted; genetic factors, posttraumatic conditions, and constitutional and behavioral factors all play a role.

Articular cartilage degeneration begins superficially, then progresses to deeper zones. As superficial chondrocytes degenerate and die, particles of fibrillated cartilage break loose into the joint. The superficial cartilage lesions fail to heal and may progress to full-thickness loss and exposed subchondral bone.

The patient is usually an athlete involved in weight training (e.g., body builder, football player) or a thrower complaining of decreased range of motion and pain. Symptoms related to loose bodies such as locking, catching, or loss of motion may be present. Examination will reveal loss of full extension and flexion and possibly decreased pronation and supination. Crepitus over the elbow and atrophy of the forearm may also be present. An effusion may be palpable over the soft spot (area bordered by the radial head, lateral condyle, and olecranon tip).

Radiographs will show the classic findings of osteoarthritis: joint space narrowing, hypertrophic spurs, and irregularity of articular surfaces. The most common areas for joint space narrowing is the radiocapitellar joint. Spurring is most frequently found about the olecranon tip, and also appears over the radial head, radial neck, and coronoid. Loose bodies may also be apparent.

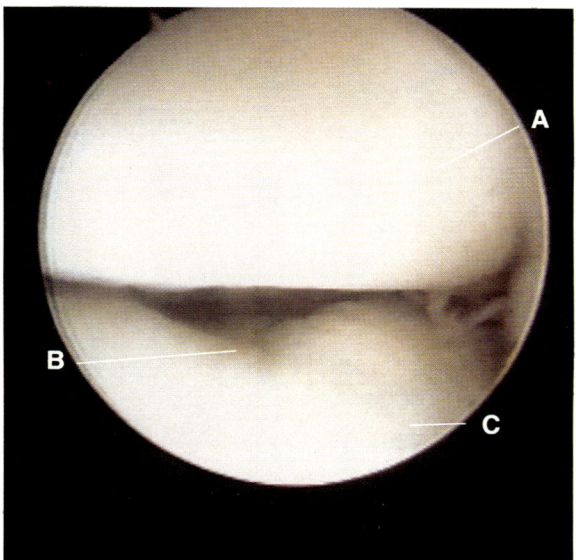

FIG 5-8. Arthroscope is in the anteromedial portal. *a*, radial head; *b*, capitellum; *c*, osteochondritis dissecans lesion of capitellum.

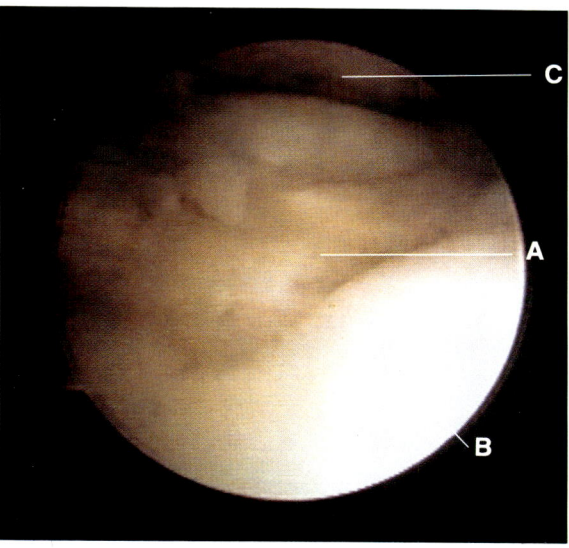

FIG 5-9. Arthroscope is in the lateral portal and the osteochondritis dissecans lesion *(a)* in the capitellum *(b)* is visible. *c*, radial head.

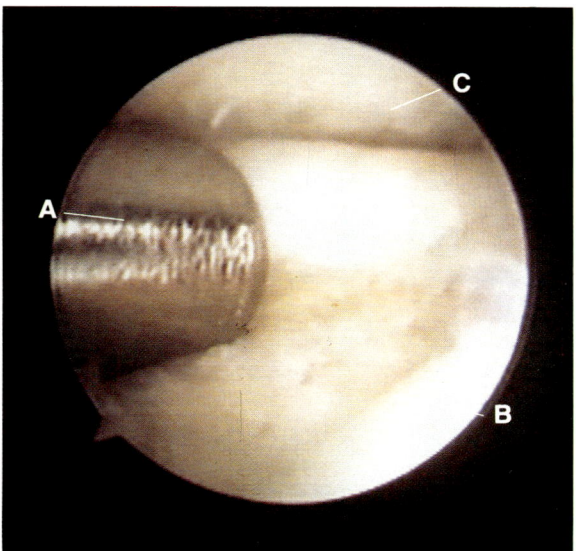

FIG 5-10. Shaver *(a)* is used through the accessory lateral portal performance of chondroplasty of the capitellum *(b)*. *c*, radial head.

68 Chapter 5

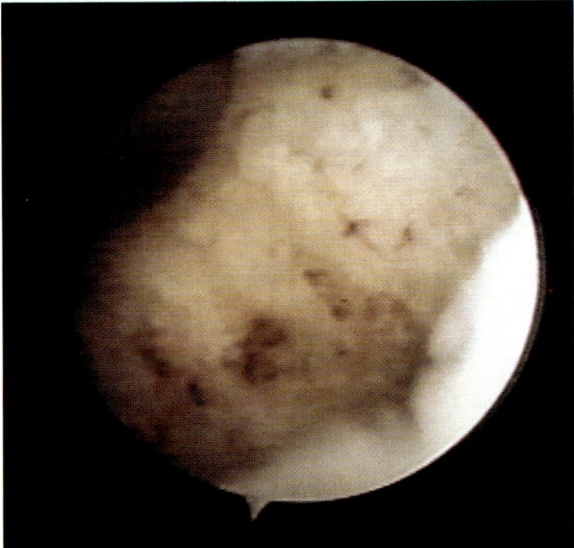

FIG 5-11. Close-up view of the base of the lesion, obtained through the lateral portal after chondroplasty-arthroplasty. Notice the bleeding bone at the base of the lesion.

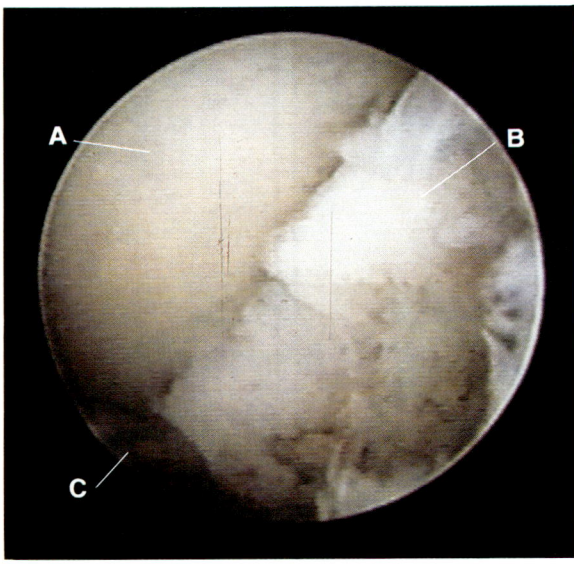

FIG 5-12. Wide-angle view obtained through the lateral portal after debridement. *a*, radial head; *b*, capitellum; *c*, shaver.

Treatment of degenerative joint disease of the elbow begins with a conservative approach. Use of antiinflammatory agents, splinting, physical therapy, and intraarticular steroid injections have been used with much success. Arthroscopic debridement and abrasion arthroplasty may be helpful when these conservative measures have failed to relieve the symptoms.

Arthroscopic abrasion arthroplasty is a modification of the original Magnusson open debridement for arthritis of the knee.[12, 15] It includes partial synovectomy, chondral shaving, osteophyte removal, loose body removal, and abrasion (i.e., drilling or burring of subchondral bone). Studies in animals and human beings have shown that multiple drill holes into subchondral bone will lead to an articular surface repair response.[8, 10, 15, 19] Newly formed tissue is reparative fibrocartilage rather than original hyaline cartilage. The successful biological and mechanical attachment of this fibrocartilage to the underlying subchondral bone correlates with improvement in symptoms.[12] One must realize that this procedure is palliative, not curative, for osteoarthritis. Contraindications to bony abrasion are inflammatory arthritis and joint instability.[14, 12]

Technique. It is imperative to measure and record flexion, extension, supination, and pronation with the patient under anesthesia, both before and after surgery, to define the goals of postoperative rehabilitation. For example, if after surgery 110 degrees of flexion is achieved with the patient under general anesthesia, this will be the ultimate goal of postoperative rehabilitation for flexion. Another important concept is to be cognizant of tourniquet time, and to proceed through each compartment without delay. In the osteoarthritic elbow, much work needs to be done in all compartments during a limited amount of time.

The techniques of partial synovectomy, chondral shaving, and loose body removal are addressed in other sections. This description will focus on osteophyte removal and abrasion of subchondral bone.

After establishment of anteromedial and anterolateral portals, the anterior compartment bony structures are evaluated. Coronoid spurs are common, as are radial head and neck osteophytes. First, synovitis is removed with the arthroscopic shaver so that visualization is improved. "Preparation before execution" is one of the basic tenets of arthroscopic surgery and has application in this situation. It is especially important to define the borders of the osteophytes so that the areas to resect can be discerned. Once this is accomplished, the surgeon uses either a ¼-inch straight osteotome or a round burr to remove spurs. If the osteotome is being used, one hand is placed on the arthroscope, one hand is used to control the osteotome, and the first assistant lightly taps the osteotome after it is placed in the proper position. One should err toward removal of more bone rather than of less because the actual size of the osteophyte tends to be underestimated. Visualization of the sharp ends of the osteotome at all times prevents injury to normal intraarticular anatomy. The osteophytic fragment is partially detached so as not to convert it to a loose body. The fragment is then removed with the arthroscopic grasper.

If too large a fragment is resected, a large hole in the capsule and skin will have to be made to remove it. This will lead to soft tissue extravasation and possible early termination of the procedure or even neurovascular injury. If a large spur exists, the surgeon resects small pieces of it at a time, to prevent this complication. After removal of the fragment, the burr is used to contour the bony edges. The coronoid fossa and radial fossa may be filled with loose bodies or hypertrophic bone that block flexion. The shaver and burr are used to debride and to reestablish the fossa so that full flexion may be achieved.

The elbow is flexed and extended, and the forearm is pronated and supinated to allow visualization of as much anatomy as possible. Evaluation for impingement, especially of the coronoid in the coronoid fossa during flexion, should be performed. One may then remove all impinging soft tissue and bone. Finally, the arthroscope is placed into the anteromedial portal to complete visualization of the entire anterior compartment.

The lateral and accessory lateral portals are established. As stated previously, synovitis should be debrided first. Usually a 3.5-mm shaver and a 2.7-mm arthroscope work best in this compartment. If subchondral bone is exposed, a 3.5-mm burr is used to abrade the superficial 1 to 2 mm of exposed bone. One need not burr deep to the subchondral bone. Abrading bone too deeply to visualize bleeding bone is a common error. Bleeding bone will usually not be seen until the inflow pump is turned off and suction is applied to the area with a shaver. Streaming of blood (bleeding bone) will then appear. The abrasion is extended to include 1 to 2 mm of adjacent cartilage. This allows soft tissue adherence of the newly formed fibrocartilage to the adjacent hyaline cartilage.[12]

The posterolateral and straight posterior (transtriceps) portals are then established. In performance of synovial debridement near medial spurs, such as in arthritic patients or patients with valgus extension overload, the surgeon must be wary of the ulnar nerve. It lies just beneath the synovium near the medial spur and may be exposed and injured during shaving or burring. The suction should be set on low or off when motorized instruments are used in this area. Use of an osteotome medially to remove olecranon spurs is safer than motorized shavers or burrs. When normal olecranon articular cartilage is seen at the olecranon tip after bone removal, spur resection is complete. The elbow is flexed and extended to evaluate for soft tissue or bony impingement, and the olecranon fossa is cleared of loose bodies or hypertrophic bone.

At the end of the procedure, the traction is removed and the elbow is manipulated. The limits of flexion and extension are measured with a sterile goniometer so that goals for postoperative rehabilitation are established. One may not always achieve full extension and flexion after debridement, because of soft tissue contractures. Anterior capsule, brachialis, or biceps contractures will limit extension, and posterior capsule or triceps contractures may limit flexion. Closed suction drainage in the anterior and the posterior compartments completes the operation.

Case History

A 17-year-old high school baseball pitcher complains of right elbow pain, morning stiffness, and loss of full flexion(Figs 5–13-5–20).

Valgus Extension Overload

As mentioned briefly above, a posteromedial osteophyte may develop in a thrower's elbow. This is secondary to valgus extension overload during the acceleration phase of pitching.[32] Secondarily, the follow-through phase may contribute to impingement posteriorly. This posteromedial osteophyte may abut into the medial margin of the olecranon fossa and create a painful area of chondromalacia.[32] Clinical presentation is usually that of a 25-year-old pitcher complaining of posterior elbow pain during acceleration and

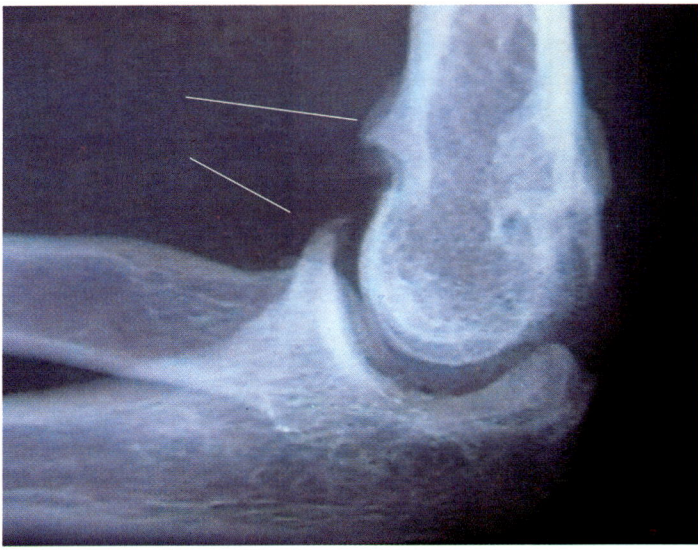

FIG 5–13. Lateral view of the right elbow shows anterior osteophytes of the coronoid and the anterior humerus.

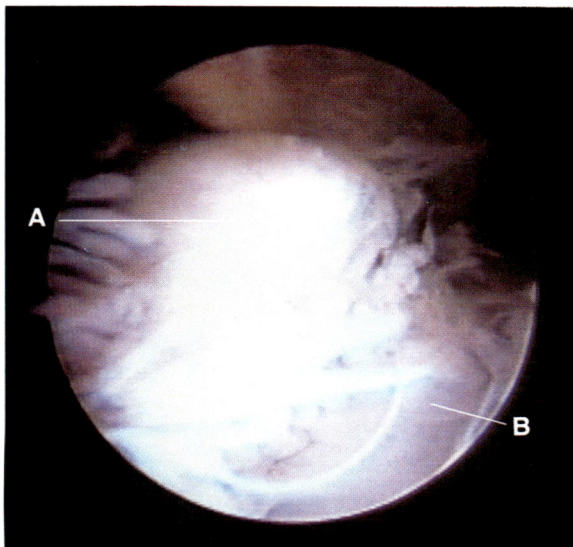

FIG 5-14. Arthroscopic view from the anterolateral portal shows osteophytes of *(a)* the anterior coronoid and *(b)* the distal humerus. As the elbow is flexed, the coronoid osteophyte impinges on the distal humeral osteophyte, which prevents full flexion.

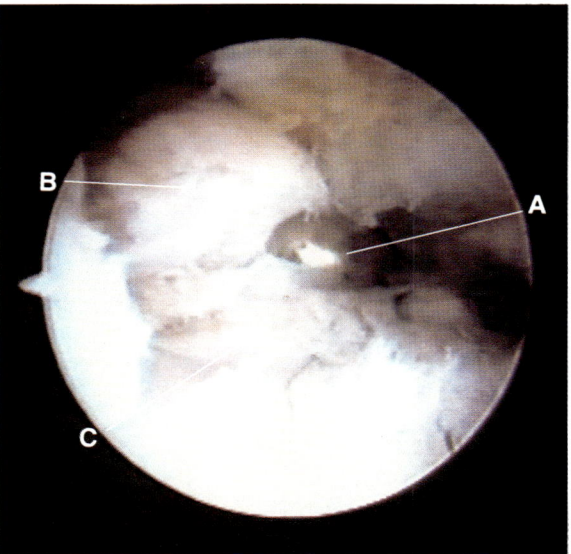

FIG 5-15. Shaver *(a)* is placed through the anteromedial portal to debride the scar tissue around the perimeter of the coronoid osteophyte *(b)*. c, distal humerus.

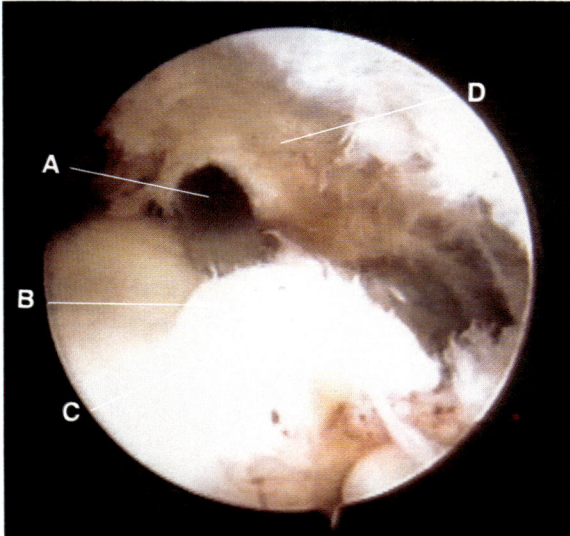

FIG 5-16. Osteotome *(a)* is placed through the anteromedial portal to remove an osteophyte *(b)* from the distal humerus *(c)*. d, medial capsule.

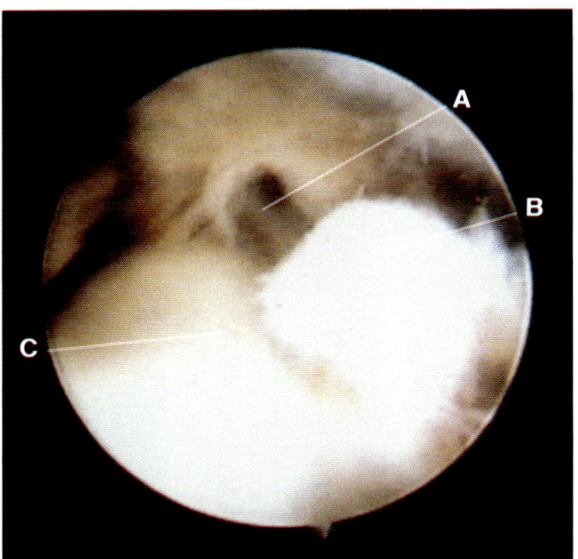

FIG 5–17. Same view shown in Figure 5-16. Osteotome *(a)* is used as a wedge to elevate the anterior osteophyte *(b)* off of the distal humerus *(c)*.

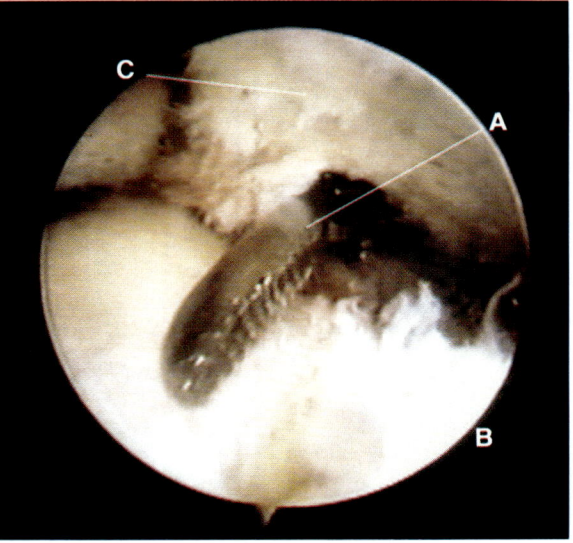

FIG 5–18. Same view shown in Figures 5-16 and 5-17. Loose body retriever *(a)*, through the anteromedial portal, is used to grasp the loose osteophyte *(b)* and remove it from the joint. *c*, medial capsule.

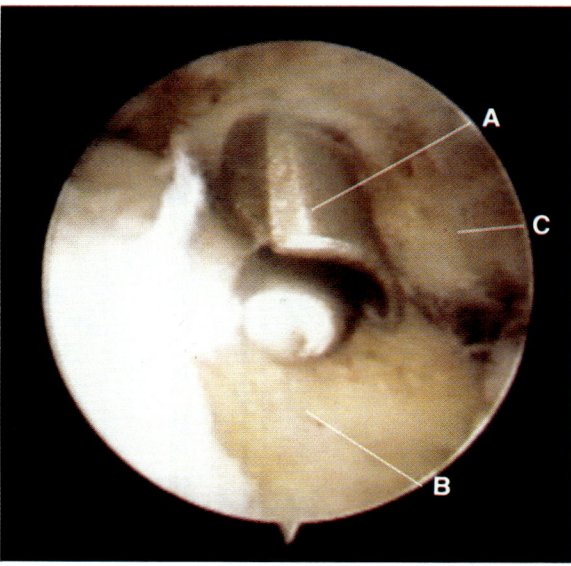

FIG 5–19. Same view shown in Figures 5-16, 5-17, and 5-18. Motorized burr *(a)* through the anteromedial portal is used to remove the base of the osteophyte *(b)*, to allow the coronoid to pass freely over this area. *c*, medial capsule.

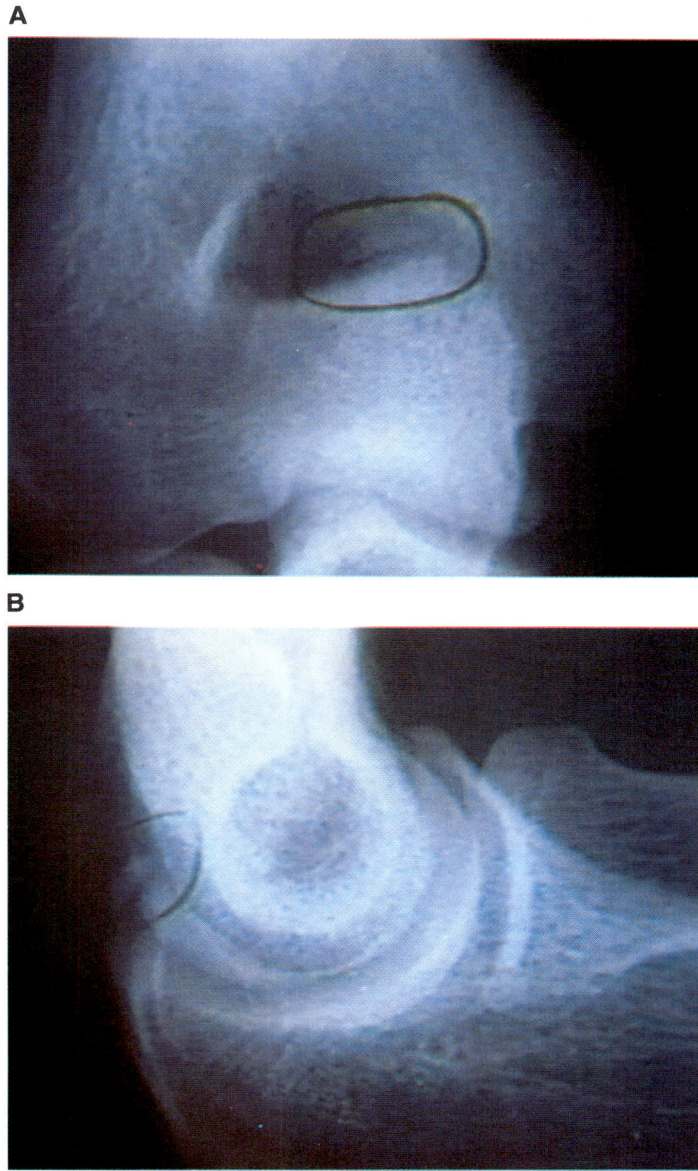

FIG 5–20. Anteroposterior (**A**) and lateral (**B**) radiographs reveal a loose body at the olecranon tip, as well as posterior impingement.

follow-through phases of pitching. Loss of ball control, with early release and high pitches, are also common complaints. Examination reveals a flexion contracture, pain over the olecranon process posteriorly, and pain with valgus stress and extension. A posterior osteophyte on the olecranon tip will be evident on the lateral radiographic view. Loose bodies associated with the olecranon tip may also be present. Axial views may show the posteromedial osteophyte.

Conservative treatment aimed at increasing strength and relieving pain initially may be used. Once a posteromedial osteophyte is present, however, symptoms will usually not be completely relieved until it is removed surgically.[32]

Technique. With the arthroscope in the posterolateral portal, resection of approximately 1 cm of the olecranon process is performed by using a ¼- or ⅛- inch osteotome via the trans-triceps portal to make a curved osteotomy into the posteromedial olecranon. The spur is removed with a grasper. An arthroscopic burr may then be used for further bony resection (see Fig 5-21). One needs to be cognizant of the close proximity of the ulnar nerve. Shavers or burrs with suction on full are dangerous in this area. There usually exists a "kissing lesion" of chondromalacia on the medial wall of the olecranon fossa. This may require debridement or abrasion depending on the depth of the lesion.

Case History

A 24-year-old professional pitcher complains of posterior elbow pain during the follow-through phase of pitching. He also complains of loss of full elbow extension (Figs 5–22-5–30).

ARTHROLYSIS FOR ELBOW CONTRACTURES

The elbow is one of the most common joints of the body to develop loss of motion. The cause is often related to trauma, but may also be the result of acquired and congenital mechanisms.[21] Dislocations and fractures may cause intraarticular and extraarticular in-

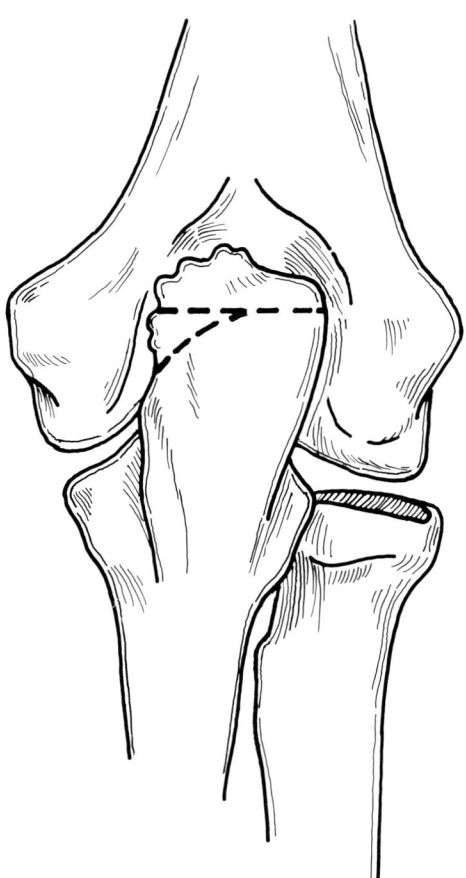

FIG 5–21. Posterior aspect of elbow. Resection of posterior olecranon tip.

Arthroscopic Surgical Procedures of the Elbow: Common Cases 75

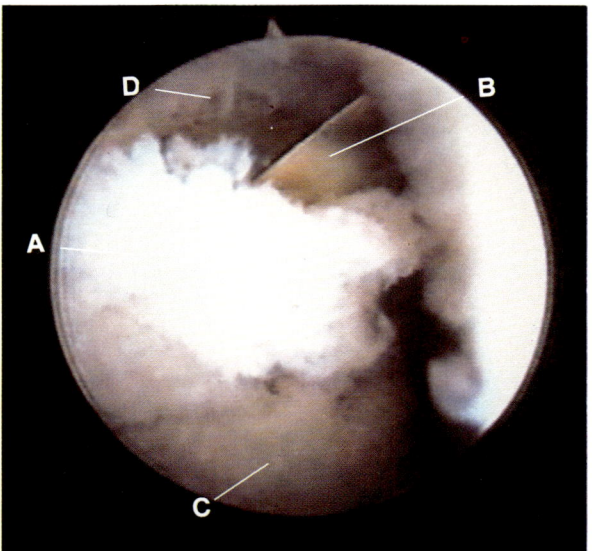

FIG 5–22. Arthroscopic view through the posterolateral portal. An arthroscopic banana knife *(b)* inserted through the straight posterior portal is used to dissect the loose body *(a)* from the olecranon *(c)* tip. *d*, humerus.

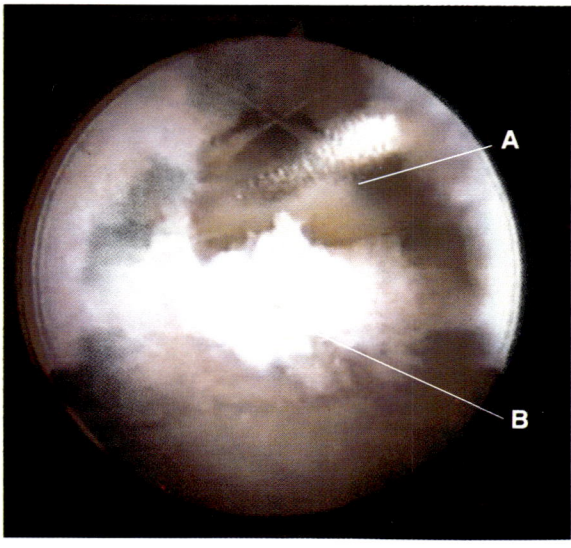

FIG 5–23. Shaver *(a)* inserted through the straight posterior portal is used to remove the loose body *(b)*.

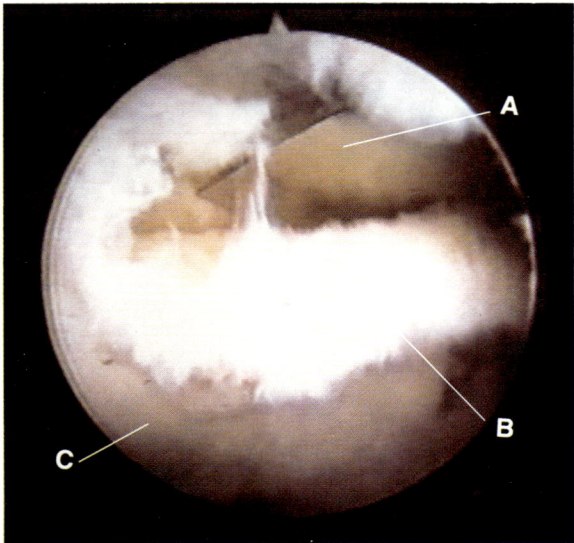

FIG 5–24. Osteotome *(a)* inserted through the straight posterior portal is used to remove a posterior osteophyte *(b)* from the olecranon tip. *c*, humerus.

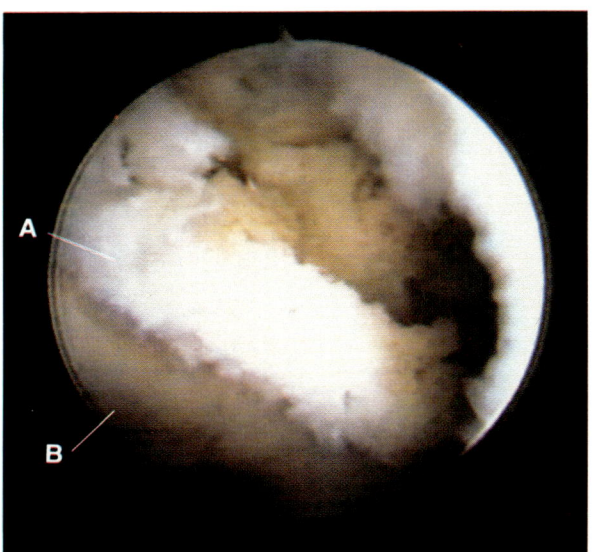

FIG 5–25. Osteophyte *(a)* is now free in the posterior compartment. *b,* humerus.

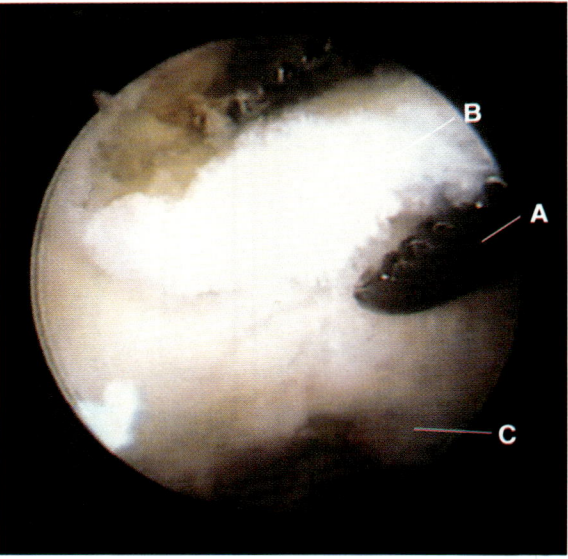

FIG 5–26. Loose body retriever *(a)* inserted through the straight posterior portal is used to remove the loosened osteophyte *(b)*. *c,* humerus.

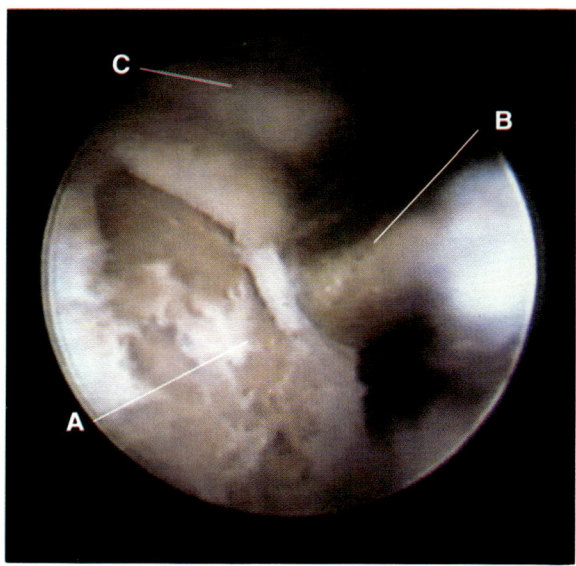

FIG 5–27. At the medial aspect of the distal humerus, a "kissing lesion" of chondromalacia *(a)* is revealed. A shaver *(b)* inserted through the straight posterior portal is being used to perform abrasion arthroplasty of the lesion. *c,* olecranon tip.

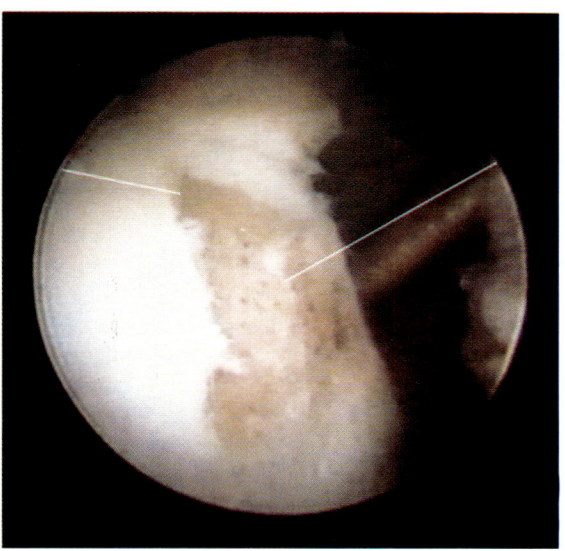

FIG 5–28. Arthroscopic view obtained after abrasion arthroplasty. The base of the lesion has punctate bleeding (left line), and the edges of lesion do not (right line).

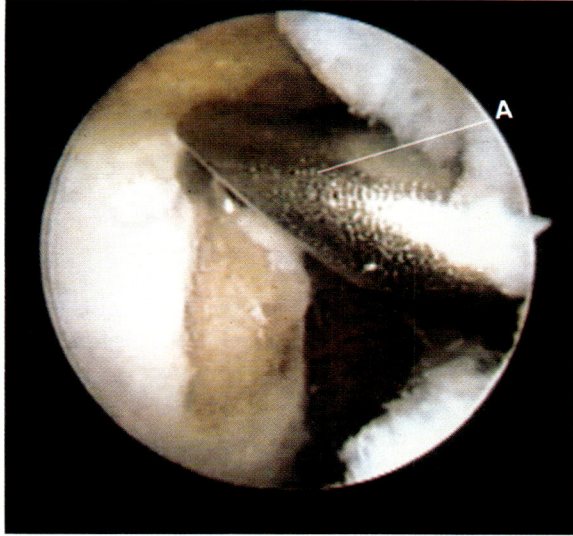

FIG 5–29. Motorized burr *(a)* inserted through the straight posterior portal is used to reduce the edges of a lesion on the humerus down to bleeding bone. The burr is also used to complete osteophyte removal from the olecranon tip.

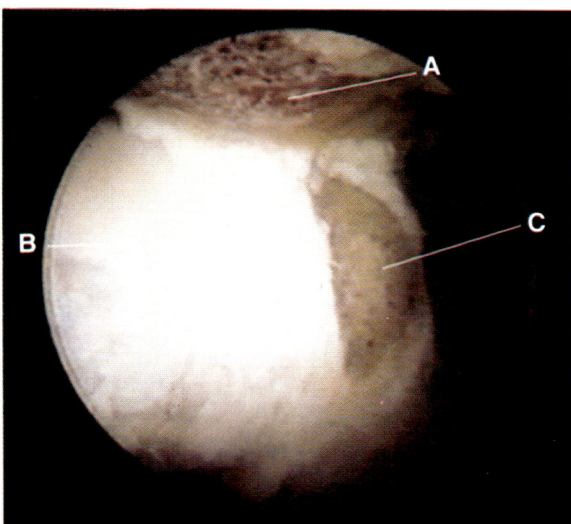

FIG 5–30. Arthroscopic view obtained after arthroscopic surgery was completed in the posterior compartment. *a*, olecranon tip; *b*, humerus; *c*, area of "kissing lesion."

jury. Periarticular soft tissues are stretched, torn, or crushed and become edematous and hemorrhagic. A hemarthrosis ensues. The elbow joint flexes in response to pain and to hemarthrosis. The periarticular soft tissues and joint capsule become shortened and fibrotic.[3, 7, 11, 21] Loss of motion may also be secondary to intraarticular causes such as malunion, osteochondral or chondral fragments, intraarticular adhesions, and loose bodies.

Nontraumatic acquired contractures may be secondary to osteoarthritis, inflammatory arthritis (e.g., rheumatoid arthritis), septic arthritis, burns, and paralysis.[21] In these conditions, the inflammation and pain lead to a flexed posture of the elbow that may become permanent. Periarticular soft tissues may become shortened and fibrotic, as with traumatic contractures. Intraarticular adhesions, synovitis, and hypertrophic osteophytes may also cause loss of motion.

The clinical presentation varies, depending on the cause of the elbow contracture. The patient will usually complain of loss of extension and flexion or both. In a throwing athlete, loss of extension is usually due to valgus extension overload, loose bodies, or injury to the anterior soft tissues (brachialis muscle or anterior capsule). Loss of motion in the thrower may be the result of osteochondritis dissecans, coronoid fossa impingement, loose bodies, or injuries to the posterior soft tissues (triceps or posterior capsule). Pronation and supination of the forearm may also be decreased. The patient may often complain of pain at the extremes of range of motion.

Standard radiography may be helpful in determinination of the exact cause of the joint contracture. Spurs, loose bodies, articular incongruity, heterotopic ossification, and joint space narrowing may be evident on plain radiographs. Tomography, CT, and MR imaging may also be indicated.

Initial treatment begins with a conservative approach. Nonsteroidal antiinflammatory medications, stretching, continuous passive motion, dynamic splinting, local application of heat, and ultrasound may be used. If this conservative approach proves inadequate, operative intervention is a treatment option.[30] We have found arthroscopic lysis of adhesions and thorough debridement to be helpful in selected cases. An elbow with severe ankylosis is a contraindication to elbow arthroscopy and is more amenable to open procedures. In mild or moderate contractures, arthroscopic surgery affords a less invasive approach than open procedures. The use of arthroscopy in treatment of contractures of the elbow is controversial; however, our experience has yielded positive results in selected patients.

Technique. Degrees of flexion, extension, supination, and pronation should be measured and recorded before surgery (before and after anesthesia) and after surgery while the patient is still anesthetized. The difference between range of motion recorded before and after anesthesia indicates the supratentorial contribution toward loss of motion in the patient. The lesser range of motion before anesthesia is usually secondary to pain. Postoperative measurements will indicate the net gain from the surgery and will serve as a guide toward the ultimate goal of postoperative therapy.

Arthroscopy in a patient with elbow contracture is challenging even to the most experienced elbow arthroscopists. It is often difficult for the surgeon to distend and gain entry into the joint space. The capsule is contracted and fibrotic. One may be unable to initially distend the joint with more than 10 or 15 mL of fluid. Penetration with a blunt trocar may be difficult, and a sharp trocar may be necessary. One must be cognizant of potential injury to neurovascular or intraarticular structures when using a sharp trocar.

The anterolateral and anteromedial portals are established in the standard fashion. Previous trauma or surgery may alter elbow anatomy. Specifically, the location of the ulnar nerve should be considered before the anteromedial portal is established.

If visualization of the localizing needle for the anteromedial portal is difficult because of intraarticular loose bodies or adhesions, the techniques described previously (see the preceding section on loose bodies) should be used to help establish this portal. The shaver is placed through the anteromedial portal to remove debris, adhesions, and synovitis to improve visualization. One assesses the anteromedial portal location and makes adjustments to obtain the ideal portal position. This may be accomplished by repuncturing the capsule under direct visualization. The arthroscope is switched into the anteromedial portal, and the anterolateral portal is similarly assessed. Once both portals are ideal, arthroscopic surgery can proceed with peak efficiency.

A shaver is used to debride the fibrotic anterior capsule from the anterior humerus. It is placed flush on bone to "peel off" the capsule from the distal humerus. This is much safer than placing the shaver directly on the anterior capsule, where neurovascular structures are anterior and endangered. Soft tissue and bone in the coronoid fossa are debrided. Medial and lateral gutters are also debrided, along with loose bodies and chondral and osseous fragments. It is helpful to use the shaver during most of this debridement. The alternative is frequent switching from shaver to banana blade to loose body grabber, which may lead to loss of the difficult-to-establish portal. Finally, the surgeon should flex and extend the elbow and rotate the forearm to complete visualization of the anterior compartment. The surgeon needs to be cognizant of the tourniquet time and to move quickly in the anterior compartment, because much work remains to be performed in the lateral, and especially, the posterior compartment. Also, throughout the procedure, frequent palpation of the anterior soft tissues for extravasation is critical. Should severe swelling or tenseness of the anterior soft tissues occur, the procedure is immediately terminated.

One now proceeds to the lateral compartment and establishes the direct lateral portal. Visualization of bony structures may be obscured by thick adhesions. An 18-gauge needle is placed 1 cm distal to the lateral portal and is directed to the tip of the arthroscope. The skin over the needle is incised, and a 3.5-mm shaver is placed through this portal and into the lateral compartment. The capitellum may be palpated with the end of the shaver, and the scar lying over it may be debrided. As the bony contours of the radiocapitellar joint appear from beneath the adhesions, debriding should continue until the joint space is free of scar. The forearm is rotated as the scar around the radial head is debrided. One should not debride distal to the radial head, because the annular ligament and the posterior interosseous nerve lie in this area. The radial recess of the ulna is also debrided of scar. The lateral aspect of the humeroulnar joint is then followed from distal to proximal, and adhesions are removed with the shaver. One may establish another accessory portal, just proximal to the direct lateral portal, to aid in this debridement. The debridement is continued until the olecranon tip is visualized.

Establishment of the posterolateral portal may be quite difficult. Much debris and synovitis is often in this area, and a direct visualization technique to establish this portal (see Chapter 4) may not be possible. This portal may be established blindly and safely, if necessary. The appropriate area for portal placement (3 cm proximal to the olecranon tip, just lateral to the triceps tendon) should be marked before arthroscopy. The skin only is incised with a no. 11 blade, and the soft tissues are spread with a hemostat. This protects the posterior antebrachial cutaneous nerve and lateral brachial cutaneous nerve from injury. A trocar is placed through this portal, aiming toward the olecranon tip. The arthroscope is introduced through the sheath. After establishment of this portal, the transtriceps portal is established under direct vision. One should err toward lateral to midline puncture, to protect the ulnar nerve, which lies medially. Debridement with a shaver through the trans-triceps portal may begin. One may need to place the shaver directly on the posterior aspect of the olecranon and peel off the posterior capsule from the bone in a similar fashion as performed anteriorly. To remove scar from the posterolateral corner, it may be helpful to place the arthroscope in the transtriceps portal and shaver in the posterolateral portal. The posteromedial debridement is performed last. The shaver is placed directly on bone with minimal, if any, suction, to avoid injury to the ulnar nerve. When debridement is complete, the range of motion should be measured with a sterile goniometer and recorded in the operative note, and drains should be placed in anterior and posterior compartments.

Case History

A 12-year-old little league catcher complains of 3 years of right lateral elbow pain and 4 to 5 months of loss of motion. Range of motion is 40 to 120 degrees (Figs 5–31-5–40).

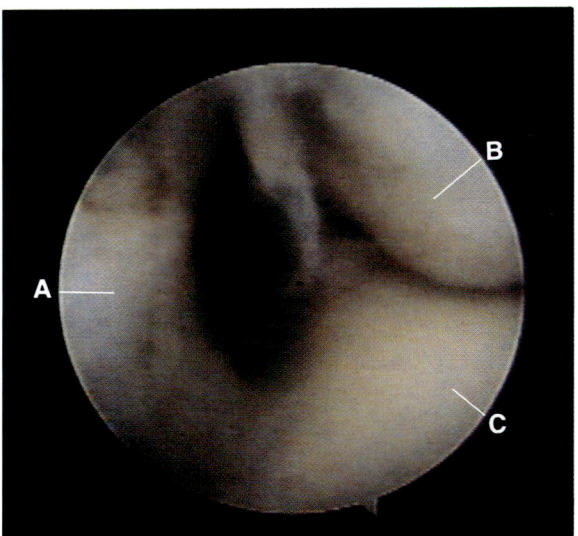

FIG 5–31. Arthroscopic view through the anteromedial portal shows large intraarticular adhesions *(a)*, coronoid *(b)*, and humerus *(c)*.

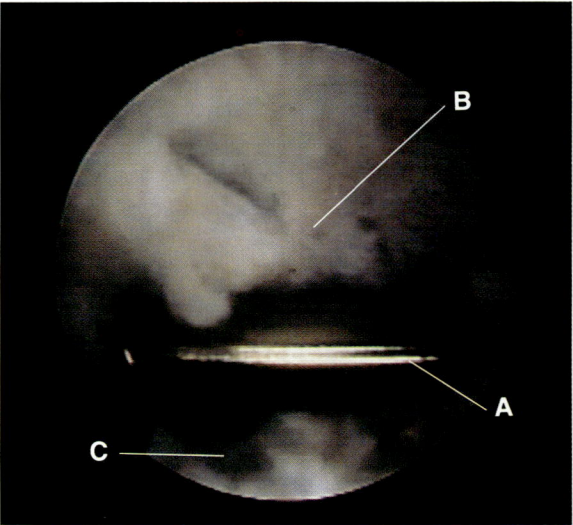

FIG 5–32. A shaver *(a)* inserted through the anterolateral portal is used to debride adhesions. *b*, hypertrophied anterior capsule; *c*, distal humerus.

Arthroscopic Surgical Procedures of the Elbow: Common Cases   81

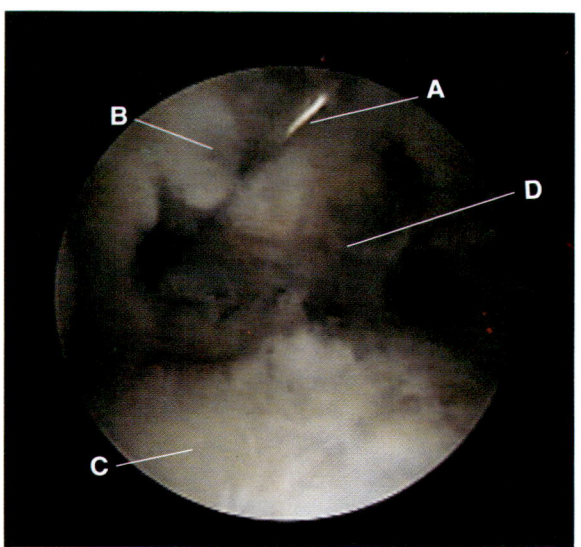

FIG 5–33. Arthroscopic knife *(a)* inserted through the anterolateral portal is used to incise adhesions in the lateral gutter *(b)*. *c*, anterior humerus; *d*, lateral capsule.

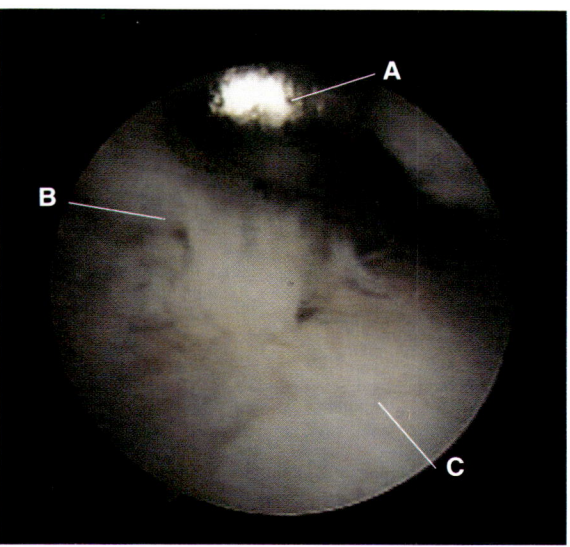

FIG 5–34. Arthroscope has been switched to the anterolateral portal. The shaver *(a)*, inserted through the anteromedial portal, removes adhesions *(b)*. C, humerus.

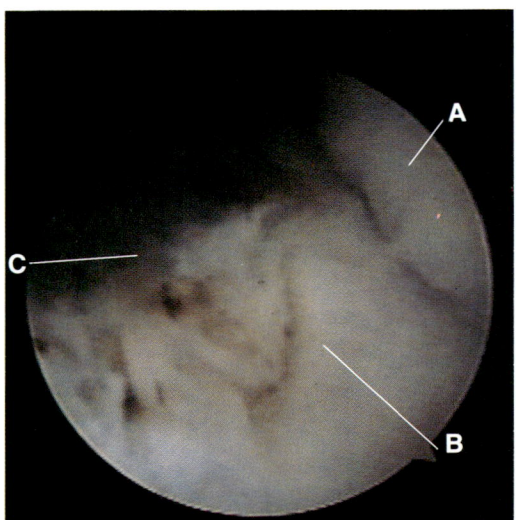

FIG 5–35. View of anterior compartment after debridement of adhesions, as seen from the anterolateral portal. *a*, coronoid; *b*, humerus; *c*, area of debridement.

82   Chapter 5

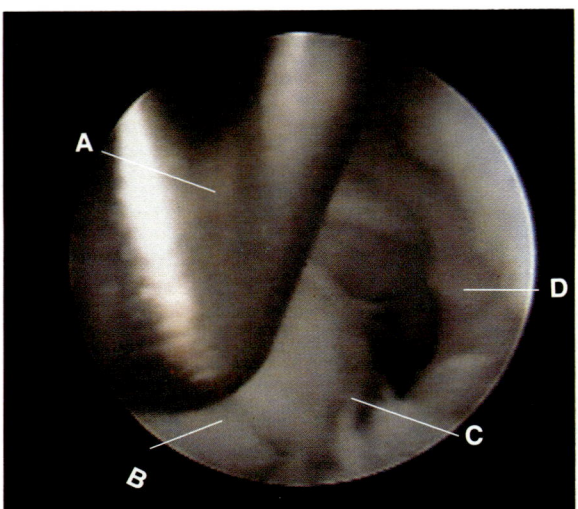

FIG 5–36. Arthroscope is in the straight lateral portal, and a shaver (a) inserted through the accessory lateral portal is used to debride adhesions (b). c, humerus; d, ulna.

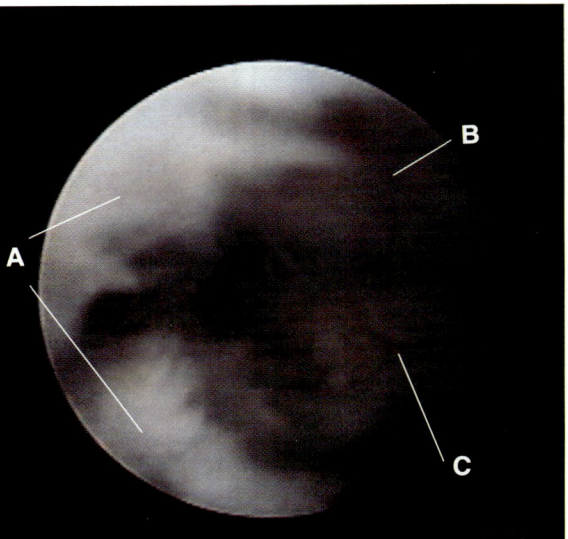

FIG 5–37. Arthroscope is in the posterolateral portal. Abundant adhesions (a) are present. b, olecranon tip; c, humerus.

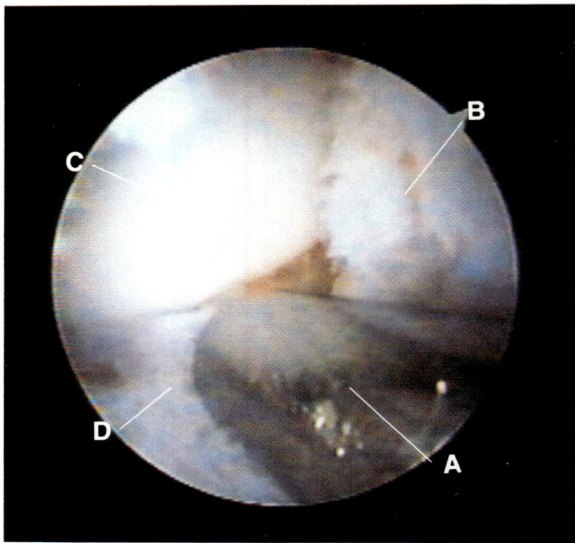

FIG 5–38. Shaver (a) inserted through the straight posterior portal is used to remove adhesions (b). c, articular surface of distal humerus.

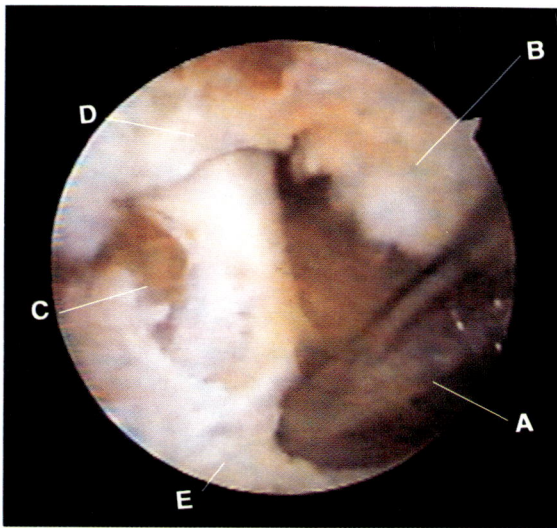

FIG 5–39. View of the posteromedial gutter. A shaver *(a)* removes adhesions *(b)*. *c*, humerus; *d*, olecranon tip.

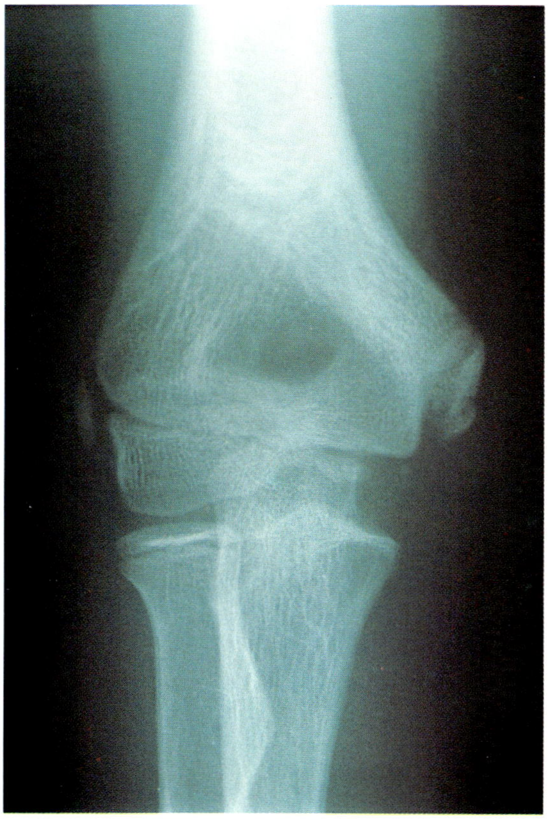

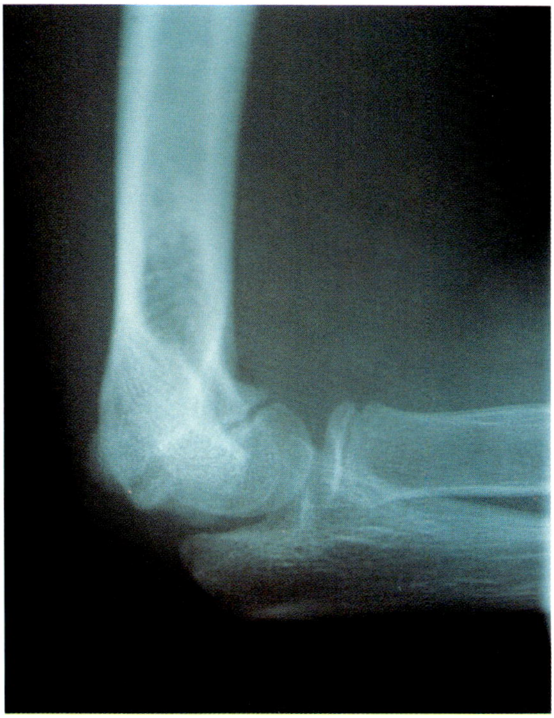

FIG 5–40. Postoperative anteroposterior **(A)** and lateral **(B)** radiographs.

EVALUATION OF ULNAR COLLATERAL LIGAMENT: ARTHROSCOPIC STRESS TEST

The most important static stabilizer to valgus elbow stress is the anterior oblique portion of the ulnar collateral ligament.[26] Acute rupture of this ligament occurs in throwing sports and in dislocations.[22, 31] Chronic valgus instability is also possible in throwing athletes, usually baseball pitchers. Stress across the medial side of the elbow during throwing may lead to an attenuation of the ulnar collateral ligament.

The clinical presentation of a patient wtih ulnar collateral ligament injury is usually that of a throwing athlete complaining of medial elbow pain during the acceleration phase of throwing. In acute rupture, a "pop" may be heard by the patient during a pitch or throw. Immediate swelling and pain ensues. Examination may reveal tenderness over the medial epicondyle, body of the ligament, or over the ulnar insertion of the ulnar collateral ligament. Ulnar nerve symptoms may be present from hemorrhage into the sheath of the ulnar nerve. Valgus stress at 15° to 20° of elbow flexion may reveal laxity; however, this is difficult to palpate, because the ulnar-humeral widening may be only a few millimeters.

Radiographic stress tests, arthrography, CT arthrography, and MR imaging, especially with saline contrast enhancement, are helpful in establishment of the diagnosis if they are positive, but even if these tests are negative, the ligament may still be lax. In this situation, arthroscopy is an excellent tool with which to evaluate the ulnar collateral

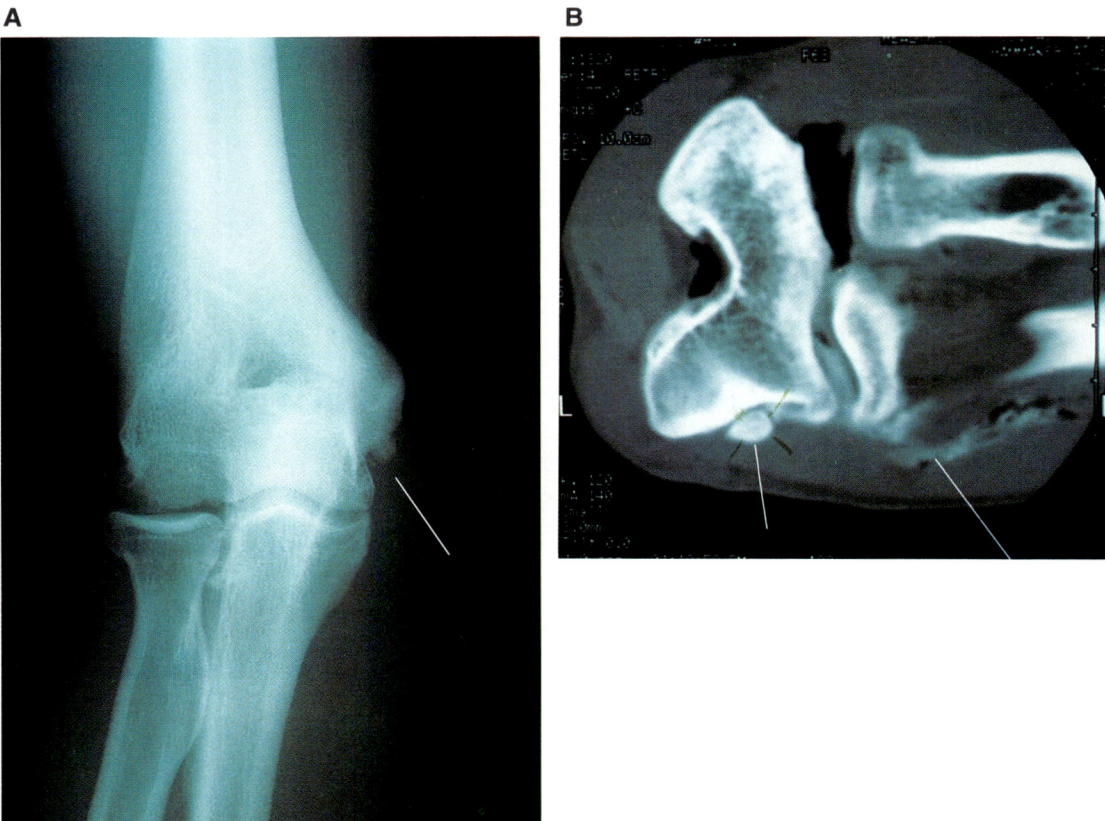

FIG 5–41. **A,** Anteroposterior radiograph and **B,** arthrographic CT scan. Left rule shows an area of previous trauma to the medial epicondyle or ulnar collateral ligament. The right rule shows leakage of contrast medium medially through an incompetent ulnar collateral ligament.

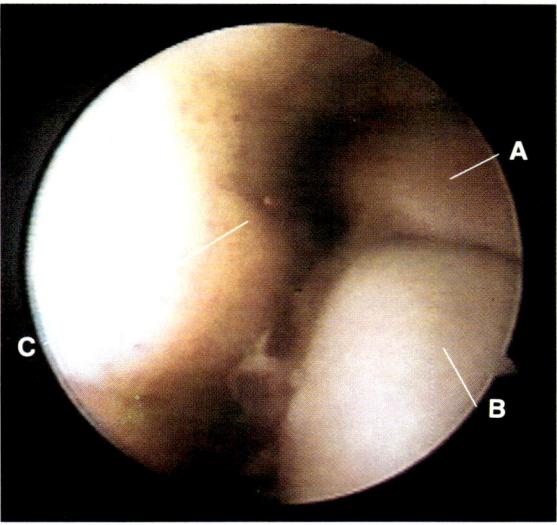

FIG 5–42. Arthroscope is in the anterolateral portal. No stress is applied to the elbow. *a*, coronoid; *b*, humerus; *c*, medial capsule.

ligament. The posterior aspect of the ulnar collateral ligament can be visualized arthroscopically (from the posterior portals), but its appearance is often normal in patients with ulnar collateral ligament laxity. The ulnar collateral ligament arthroscopic stress test[28] is a reliable and accurate means with which to assess this ligament.

Technique. With the arthroscope in the anterolateral portal, the medial aspect of the ulnar humeral joint is visualized. Traction is removed, and valgus stress at 30° of elbow flexion is applied. In the normal elbow, there will be up to 1 mm of widening of the ulnar humeral joint with this maneuver. With ulnar collateral ligament insufficiency, 2 to 10 mm of ulnar humeral opening can usually be demonstrated. Also, the posterior band of the ligament may be evaluated from the posterior compartment. With the arthroscope in the posterolateral portal, the most medial and distal aspects of the joint are visualized. The posterior band of the ulnar collateral ligament may be seen. In acute ruptures or synovitis in this region, and with chronic ulnar collateral ligament attenuation, tearing of the ligament may be seen.

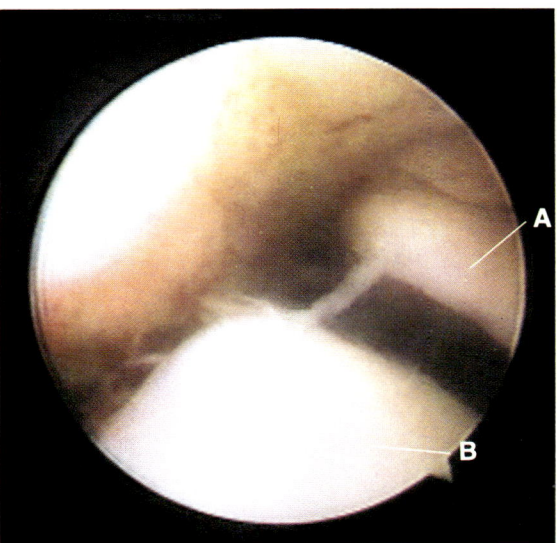

FIG 5–43. Valgus stress is applied to the elbow. Coronoid *(a)* displaces from the humerus *(b)* by several millimeters. In a normal elbow with a competent ulnar collateral ligament, minimal or no displacement occurs with valgus stress.

Case History

A 21-year-old professional pitcher complains of pain over the medial aspect of the right elbow during the acceleration phase of throwing (Figs 5–41-5–43).

REFERENCES

1. Bell MS: Loose bodies in the elbow, *Br J Surg* 62:921, 1975.
2. Boe S: Arthroscopy of the elbow: diagnosis and extraction of loose bodies, *Acta Orthop Scand* 57:52, 1986.
3. Buxton JD: Ossification in the ligaments of the elbow, *J Bone Joint Surg* 20:79, 1938.
4. Chandler EJ: Abrasion arthroplasty of the knee, *Contemp Orthop* 11:21, 1985.
5. Chiroff RT, Cooke CP: Osteochondritis dissecans: a histological and micro-radiographic analysis of surgically excised lesions, *J Trauma* 15:689, 1975.
6. Gardiner TB: Osteochondritis dissecans in three members of one family, *J Bone Joint Surg* 37B:139, 1955.
7. Green DP, McCoy H: Turnbuckle orthotic correction of elbow flexion contractures after acute injuries, *J Bone Joint Surg [Am]* 61:1092, 1979.
8. Haggart GE: The surgical treatment of DJD of the knee. *J Bone Joint Surg* 22:717, 1940.
9. Haraldsson S: An osteochondrosis deformans juvenilis capituli humeri including investigation of intraosteovasculature in distal humeras, *Acta Orthop Scand* 38(suppl):1, 1959.
10. Insall J: The Pridie debridement operation for osteoarthritis of the knee, *Clin Orthop* 101:61, 1974.
11. Johanson O: Capsular and ligament of the elbow joint: clinical and arthographic study, *Acta Chir Scand* 287(suppl):124, 1962.
12. Johnson LL: Arthroscopy abrasion arthroplasty: historical and pathologic prospectives—present status, *Arthroscopy* 2:54, 1986.
13. Konig F:Über freie Körper in den Gelenken. *Dtsc Z Chir* 27:90, 1888.
14. Larson RL, et al: Little league survey: the Eugene study, *Am J Sports Med* 4:204, 1976.
15. Magnusson PB: Joint debridement: surgical treatment of degenerative arthritis, *Surg Gynecol Obstet* 73:1, 1941.
16. McManama GD, et al. The surgical treatment of osteochondritis of the capitellum, *Am J Sports Med* 13:11, 1985.
17. Milgram JW: The classification of loose bodies in human joints, *Clin Orthop* 124:282, 1977.
18. Milgram JW: The development of loose bodies in human joints, *Clin Orthop* 124:292, 1977.
19. Mitchel N, et al: The resurfacing of adult rabbit articular cartilage by multiple perforations through the subchondral bone, *J Bone Joint Surg [Am]* 58:230, 1976.
20. Mitsunaga MM, et al: Osteochondritis dissecans of the capitellum, *J Trauma* 22:53, 1982.
21. Morrey BF: *The elbow and its disorders,* Philadelphia, 1985, WB Saunders.
22. Norwood LA, Shook JA, Andrews JR: Acute medial elbow ruptures, *Am J Sports Med* 9:16, 1981.
23. Omer GEJ: Primary articular osteochondrosis, *Clin Orthop* 158:33, 1981.
24. Pappas AM: Osteochondrosis dissecans, *Clin Orthop* 158:59, 1981.
25. Ruch DS, Poehling GG: Arthroscopic treatment of Panner's disease, *Clin Sports Med* 10:629, 1991.
26. Schwab GH, et al: Biomechanics of elbow instability: the role of the medial collateral ligament, *Clin Orthop* 146:42–52, 1980.
27. Singer KM, Roy SP: Osteochondrosis of the humeral capitellum, *Am J Sports Med* 12:351, 1984.
28. Soffer SR, Andrews JR: The ulnar collateral ligament arthroscopic stress test, in press.
29. Tullos HS, King JW: Lesions of the pitching arm in adolescence, *Trauma* 220:264, 1972.
30. Urbaniak JR, et al: Correction of post-traumatic flexion contracture of the elbow by anterior capsulotomy, *J Bone Joint Surg [Am]* 67:1160, 1985.
31. Waris W: Elbow injuries in javelin throwers, *Acta Chir Scand* 93:563, 1946.
32. Wilson FD, et al: Valgus extension overload in the pitching elbow, *Am J Sports Med* 11:83, 1983.
33. Woodward AH, Bianco AJ: Osteochondritis dissecans of the elbow, *Clin Orthop* 110:35, 1975.

Chapter 6

Arthroscopic Surgical Procedures of the Elbow: Uncommon Cases

Stephen R. Soffer, M.D.
James R. Andrews, M.D.

RHEUMATOID ARTHRITIS: SYNOVIAL BIOPSY AND SYNOVECTOMY

Approximately 20% to 50% of patients with rheumatoid arthritis have elbow involvement[1, 17, 18]; of these, 50% will have moderate to severe pain.[1] There is usually a loss of motion ranging from 30 to 50 degrees of flexion or extension and 20 to 30 degrees of forearm supination or pronation. Radiographic findings include osteopenia, effusion, narrowing of joint space, bone erosion, cystic changes, subluxation, dislocation, and angular or rotational deformity.

The mainstay of treatment is a conservative approach involving patient education, administration of oral antiinflammatory agents, physical therapy, splinting, and intraarticular injections of corticosteroids. When conservative measures fail, operative intervention may be helpful. Early synovectomy of an intact but painful rheumatoid elbow may temporarily slow its degeneration.[1] Porter et al.[17] reported pain relief in most rheumatoid patients for at least 6 years after open elbow synovectomy. Arthroscopic partial synovectomy may be of use in ameliorating the symptoms of pain in rheumatoid patients. It may not be expected to have a long-lasting effect on range of motion. Arthroscopic synovectomy, however, is more advantageous than open surgical synovectomy in that it is a less invasive procedure with less postoperative morbidity.

Technique

It is usually not difficult to perform arthroscopy in a rheumatoid elbow. The synovial joint is quite enlarged and already distended with synovial fluid, which allows easy joint entry with the trocar. The ligaments are often lax, and the arthroscope moves with ease from compartment to compartment. In fact, the arthroscopist will be able to place the arthroscope in spaces and areas that would not be accessible in a normal elbow. For example, with the arthroscope in the lateral portal, one may be able to place the arthroscope through the radiocapitellar joint and into the anterior compartment. At times, hypertrophied synovium may obscure visualization, necessitating resection.

In performance of synovial biopsy, an area of synovium that appears the most diseased should be chosen. The biopsy specimen is removed as atraumatically as possible by using a banana blade, then a grasper. The grasper must be used gently, because it may crush the specimen. Several samples are taken from different locations.

For synovectomy, anterolateral and anteromedial portals are established in standard fashion. All visible synovium is debrided with a shaver. One needs to be wary of anterior synovial shaving; the neurovascular bundle lies anterior to the synovium. The arthroscope is placed in the anterolateral portal, then the anteromedial portal, to evaluate the entire anterior compartment. By using the shaver in each of the two portals, synovectomy is completed.

In the lateral compartment, any synovium evident is debrided. The arthroscope and shaver are each placed in the accessory lateral and the direct lateral portal to complete visualization and synovectomy in this compartment.

In the posterior compartment, the synovium is debrided posterolaterally and posteriorly first, by using arthroscope and shaver in each portal. The surgeon should then debride posteromedially by using low suction, but with wariness, for the shaver is being used in close proximity to the ulnar nerve. Minimal debridement is performed in this area.

Case 1: Rheumatoid Arthritis

A 65-year-old man has a 1-year history of right elbow pain, swelling, and catching. Symptoms are aggravated during golf, especially during terminal extension and flexion motions. Examination reveals a range of motion of 10 to 120 degrees in the flexion arc, and a large effusion. Testing for rheumatoid factor gives positive results, and radiographs are normal (Figs 6–1-6–11).

TUMOR TREATMENT

Synovial Osteochondromatosis

Synovial osteochondromatosis is a benign tumor of the synovium characterized by multiple osteocartilaginous and cartilaginous nodules or loose bodies.[12, 21] The synovium

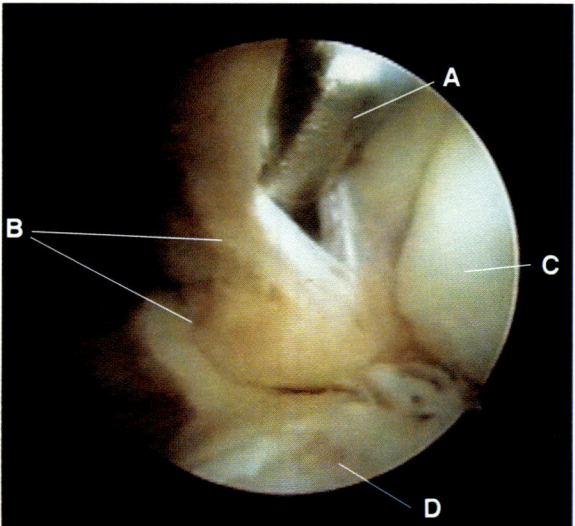

FIG 6–1. The arthroscope is in the anterolateral portal, and a shaver *(a)* inserted through the anteromedial portal is used to remove hypertrophic synovium *(b)*. *c,* coronoid, *d,* humerus.

Arthroscopic Surgical Procedures of the Elbow: Uncommon Cases 89

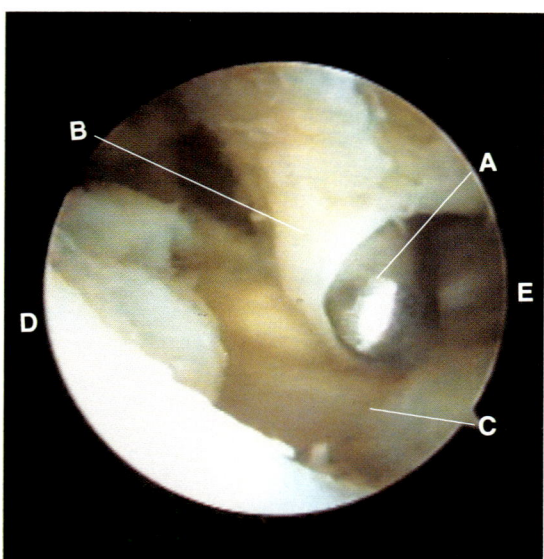

FIG 6–2. The arthroscope is in the anterolateral portal, and the shaver *(a)* is used to debride synovium *(b)* from the anterior compartment. *c*, anterior humerus, *d*, proximal, *e*, distal.

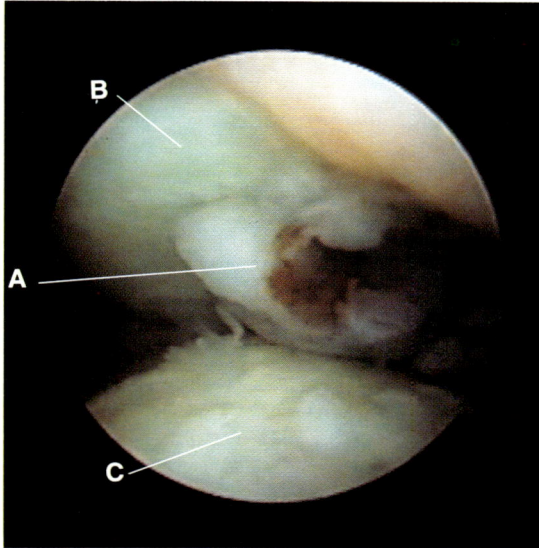

FIG 6–3. Hypertrophic synovium *(a)* is lodged between the radial head *(b)* and the capitellum *(c)*.

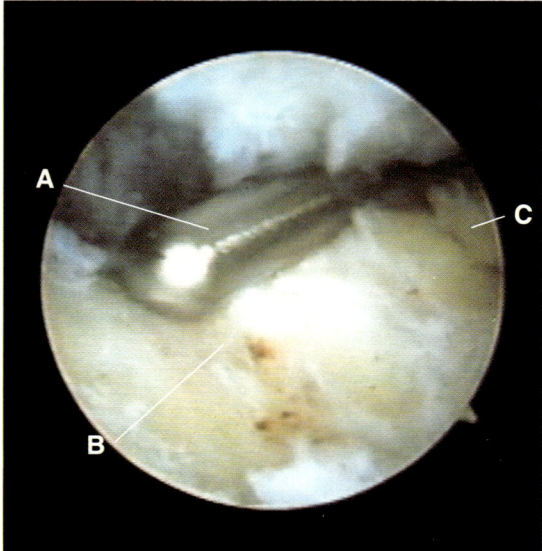

FIG 6–4. A shaver *(a)* is used to debride the coronoid fossa *(b)* of synovium. *c*, coronoid.

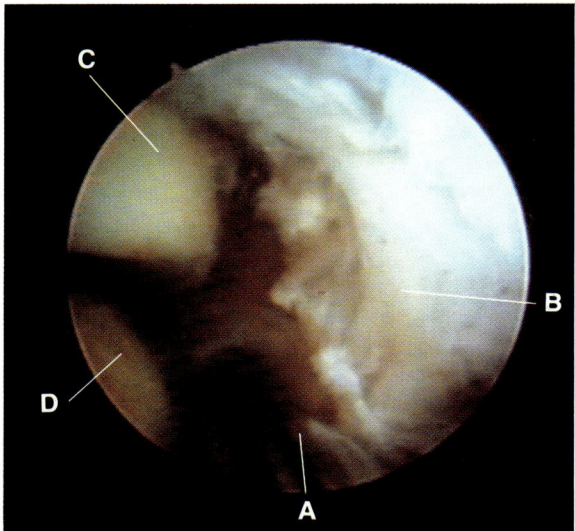

FIG 6–5. The arthroscope is in the anteromedial portal, and a shaver *(a)* inserted through the anterolateral portal is used to debride synovium *(b)*. *c,* radial head, *d,* capitellum.

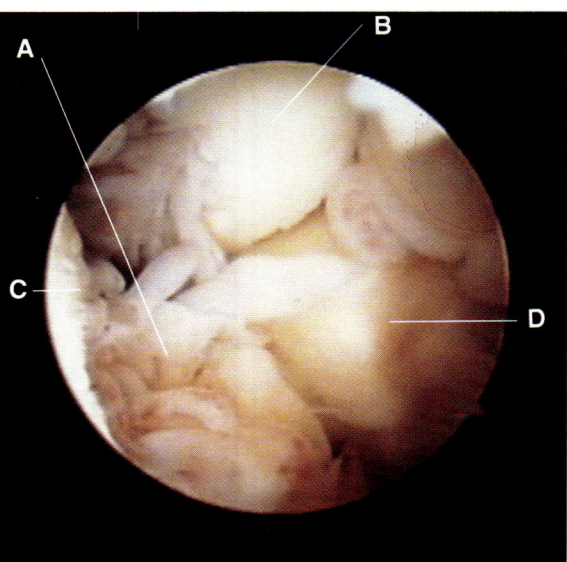

FIG 6–6. The arthroscope is in the direct lateral portal. The lateral compartment is filled with hypertrophic synovium *(a)*. *b,* radial head, *c,* capitellum, *d,* ulna.

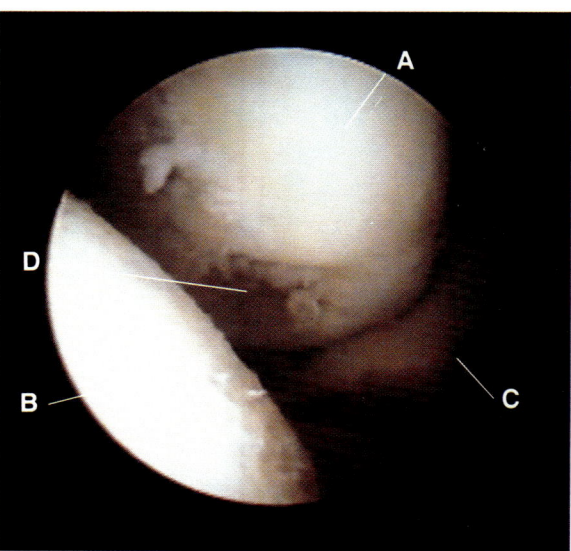

FIG 6–7. View of lateral compartment after synovectomy, showing radial head **(a)**, capitellum **(b)**, and ulna **(c)**. An osteochondral defect **(d)** created by eroding synovium is also evident.

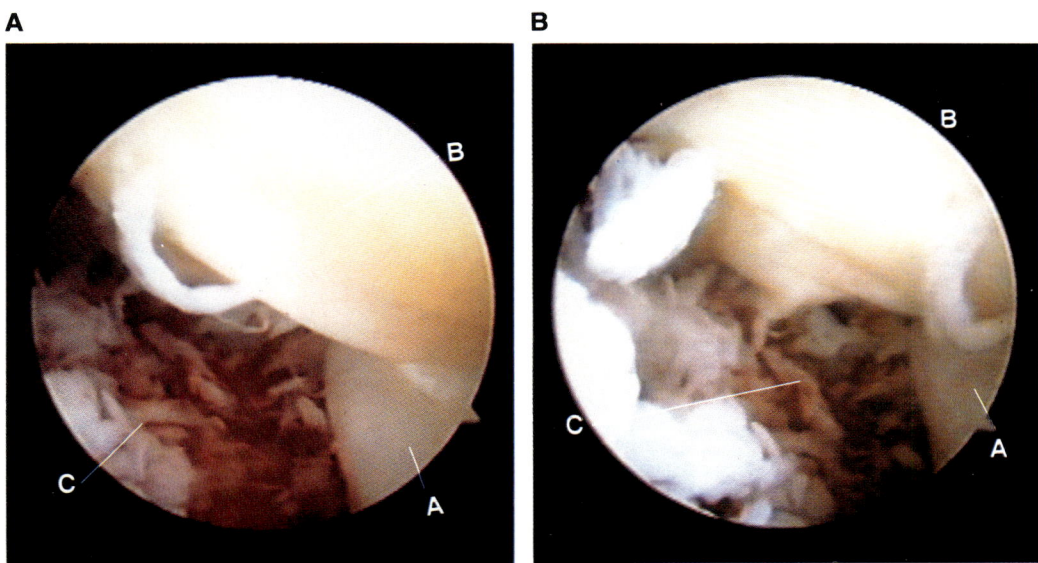

FIG 6-8. Views of the posterior aspect, with the arthroscope in the lateral compartment. *a*, ulna; *b*, humerus; *c*, synovitis.

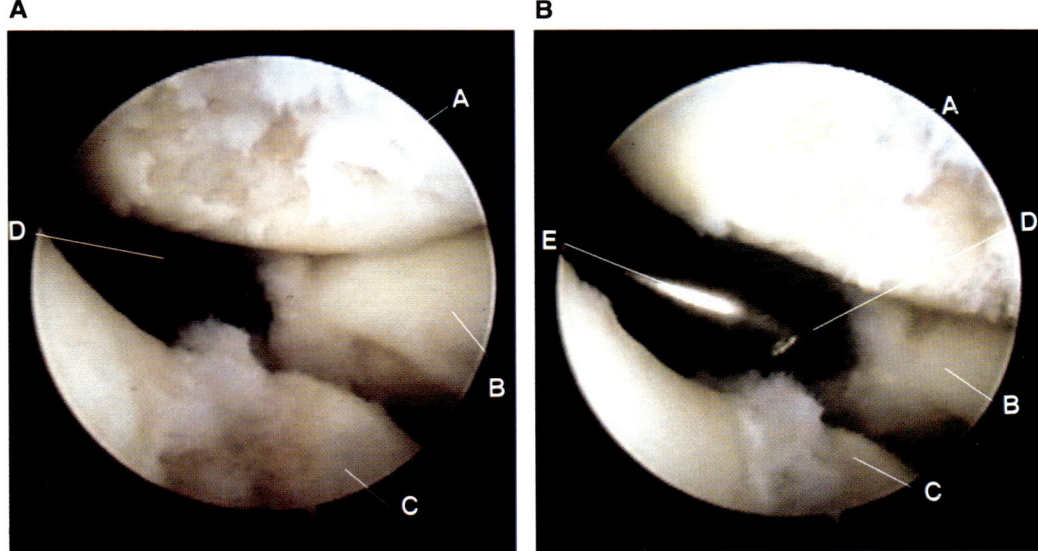

FIG 6-9. With the arthroscope in the lateral portal, the anterior compartment can be visualized because of elbow laxity. *a*, radial head; *b*, ulna; *c*, humerus; *d*, anterior compartment; *e*, cannula in anterior medial portal in anterior compartment.

undergoes metaplastic differentiation into cartilaginous tissue.[9] After the knee joint, the elbow is the second most common sight of involvement.[21]

A typical case usually involves a 40-year-old man with pain, loss of motion, and swelling. Radiographs may show opacities or no abnormality, especially in early stages of chondromatosis. Arthrography, magnetic resonance imaging, or computed tomography may show multiple loose bodies. The diagnosis is made through histologic evaluation of biopsy specimens.

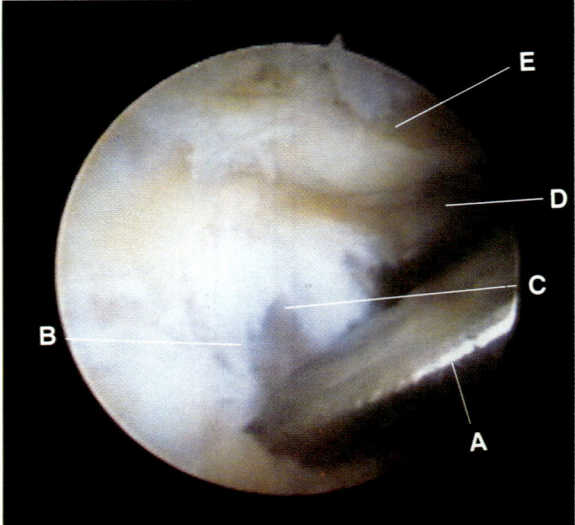

FIG 6–10. With the arthroscope in the posterolateral portal, a shaver (a) inserted through the straight posterior portal is used to debride synovium (b) from the posterior aspect of the humerus (c). d, ulna-humeral articulation; e, ulna.

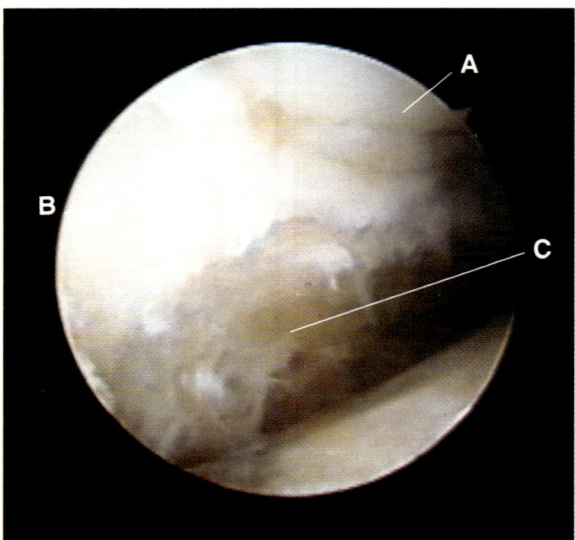

FIG 6–11. View of posterior compartment after synovectomy. a, ulna; b, humerus; c, area of debridement on posterior aspect of humerus.

Treatment involves removing loose bodies and performing synovectomy. Synovectomy may be performed by using open or arthroscopic approaches. Chondromatosis frequently recurs because of remaining synovium within the elbow joint. Thus, the arthroscopic approach has the advantage of being less invasive than open surgery, and it may be repeated with lower morbidity than with a second open surgical procedure. Secondary osteoarthritis is common in osteochondromatosis, mostly because of three-body wear from loose bodies.

Technique. After establishment of anterolateral and anteromedial portals, preliminary diagnosis of osteochondromatosis may often be made from the gross appearance of the synovium. The synovium is hyperemic, thickened, and villous. Small white nodules of cartilage or cartilage and bone are attached to the synovium in a pedunculated fashion. All or only part of the synovium may be involved. Therefore, all compartments must be evaluated for tumor. Removal of loose bodies and synovectomy are performed as described previously.

There is often a nidus of synovium in which a large concentration of budding cartilaginous bodies exist. This area must be sought diligently, and all nodules and synovium must be removed to prevent recurrence.

Case 2: Synovial Osteochondromatosis

A 56-year-old man complains of the gradual onset of pain, catching, and loss of full right elbow extension. He had undergone arthrotomy 2 years previously for removal of multiple loose bodies. Findings revealed synovial osteochondromatosis. The present range of motion is from 35 degrees to 120 degrees in the flexion arc (Figs 6–12-6–19).

Pigmented Villonodular Synovitis

Pigmented villonodular synovitis is a benign aggressive tumor of the synovium that forms villous and nodular yellow-brown projections.[21] Recently, it has been suggested that this is a reactive inflammatory process rather than a true neoplasm.[19] It rarely occurs in the elbow. Clinical presentation usually involves a young adult complaining of swelling, pain, and decreased range of motion. Examination may show joint effusion. Radiography may reveal surface erosions and cysts on both sides of the elbow joint, with no joint

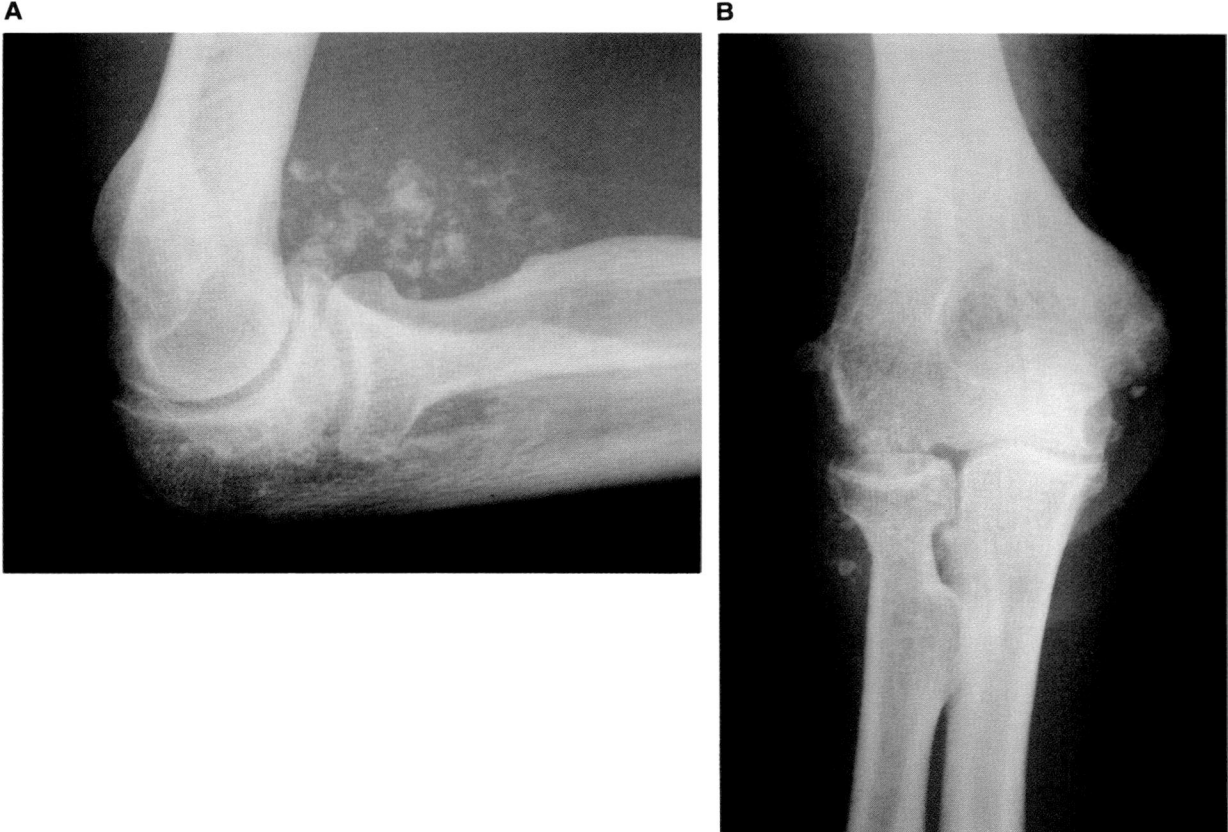

FIG 6–12. **A,** Lateral and **B,** anteroposterior radiographs show multiple loose bodies along with narrowing of joint space and early osteoarthritic changes.

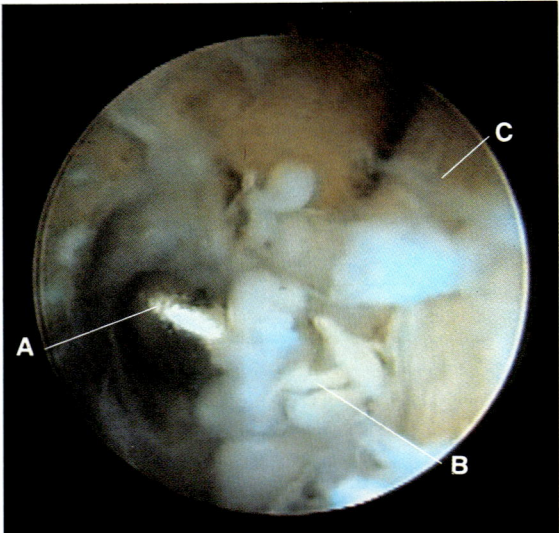

FIG 6–13. The arthroscope is in the anterolateral portal. A shaver *(a)* inserted through the anteromedial portal removes synovium and loose bodies *(b)*. *c*, coronoid.

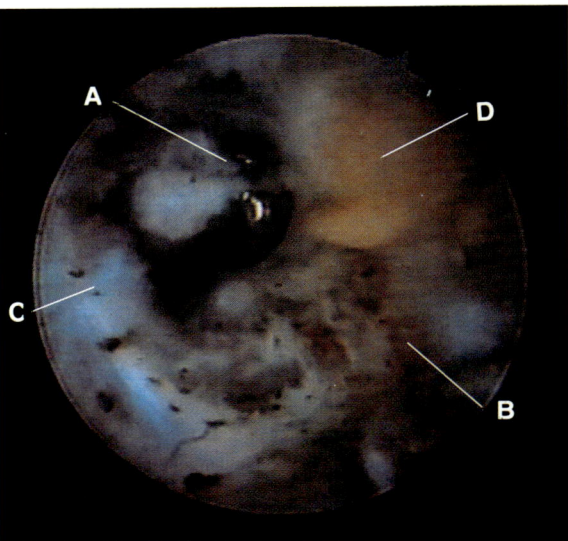

FIG 6–14. A loose body retriever (a) in the anteromedial portal is used to remove an osteochondroma. *b*, humerus; *c*, anteromedial capsule; *d*, coronoid.

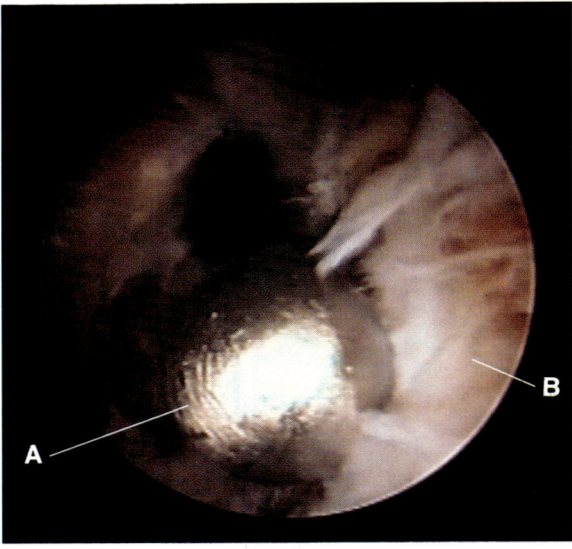

FIG 6–15. Synovectomy of the anterior compartment is performed with a shaver *(a)*. *b*, anterior humerus.

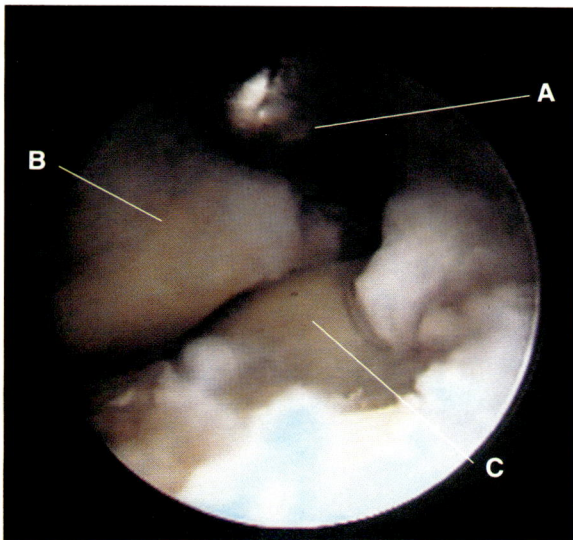

FIG 6–16. The arthroscope is in anteromedial portal, and a shaver *(a)* inserted through the anterolateral portal is used to remove chondromas from radial head *(b)*. *c*, capitellum.

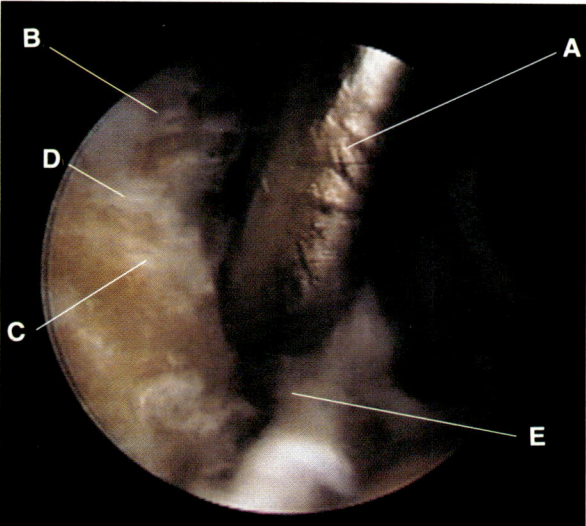

FIG 6–17. The arthroscope is in the posterolateral portal. A shaver *(a)* inserted through the straight posterior portal is used to debride synovium from the posteromedial gutter. *b*, olecranon; *c*, medial aspect of posterior humerus; *d*, ulnahumeral articulation; *e*, posteromedial gutter.

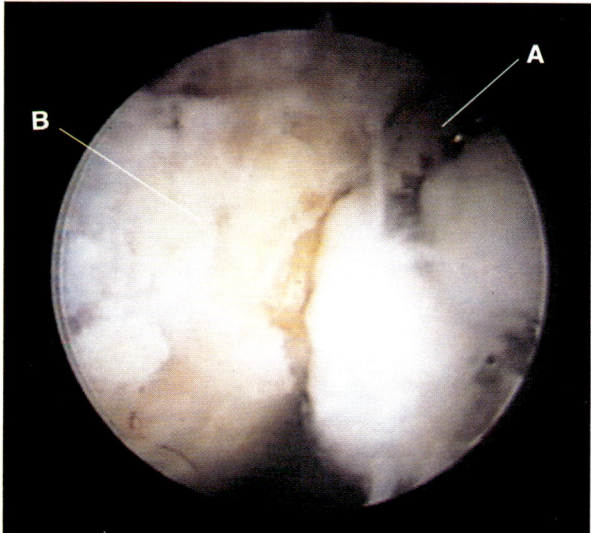

FIG 6–18. A grasper *(a)* in the straight posterior portal is used to remove loose body in the posterior compartment. *b*, humerus.

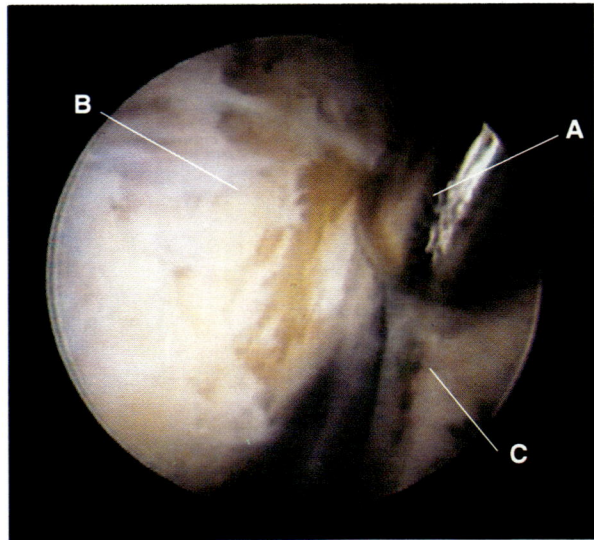

FIG 6–19. A shaver *(a)* inserted through the straight posterior portal is used to debride synovium in the posterior compartment, to prevent recurrences. *b*, humerus; *c*, posterior capsule.

space narrowing, or osteopenia, as seen in rheumatoid arthritis.[13] A soft tissue mass may also be evident on radiographs. A diagnosis is made through gross and histologic evaluation of the synovial tissue. Treatment involves excision and synovectomy. As with osteochondromatosis, there is a high recurrence rate because of the difficulty of achieving a complete synovectomy. Arthroscopic synovectomy through multiple portals is advantageous in that it provides access to all compartments of the elbow with minimal morbidity.

Technique. With the arthroscope in the anterolateral portal, one will note dark brown serosanguineous fluid and similar discoloration of the synovium. Synovial villi are hypertrophic, commonly elongated, and nodular. Synovium eroding into bone may be seen. Partial synovectomy is then performed (see section on partial synovectomy, p. 87–88).

SYNOVIAL PLICAE EXCISION

Just as synovial plicae of the knee may become fibrotic or synovitic and cause symptoms, so may plicae of the elbow. Synovial plicae are probably embryologic septal remnants. The lateral plica originates in the lateral gutter, crosses the radiocapitellar joint anteriorly and inserts onto the anterior elbow capsule.[3] It is associated with chondromalacia of the margin of the articular surface of the radial head. Clarke[3] likened these changes to those seen on the medial femoral condyle from symptomatic medial plicae of the knee. Histologic evaluation of the pathologic plicae in the Clarke series revealed synovitis and fibrosis. It is possible that lateral elbow plicae become symptomatic secondary to acute trauma or repetitive microtrauma.[3, 4]

Patients usually have catching, sharp pain, clicking, and locking. Results of examination may be normal or may reveal decreased range of motion and a popping sensation that is palpable over the radial head during flexion and pronation. Radiographs usually show no abnormality. If initial conservative treatment fails, arthroscopy with excision of the plica or synovitis may be curative.

In some patients performing repetitive extension and pronation of the forearm (such as a tennis player during the serving motion), chronic synovitis may occur in the lateral compartment. This hypertrophic synovium causes a painful snapping sensation laterally. Arthroscopic removal of this synovium is usually curative.

Technique. Anterolateral and anteromedial portals are established. With the arthroscope in the anterolateral portal, the lateral plicae is excised by using a banana blade, basket forceps, or shaver through the anteromedial portal. The surgeon must be certain to perform complete diagnostic elbow arthroscopy of the lateral and posterior compartments to rule out other diagnoses such as loose bodies, osteochondritis of the capitellum or radial head, and chondromalacia of the lateral compartment.

Case 3: Synovial Plicae

A 16-year old tennis player complains of right lateral elbow discomfort and a catching sensation while serving. Examination reveals a small effusion and tenderness over the radiocapitellar joint with palpation. Radiographs show no abnormalities (Fig 6–20).

TREATMENT OF SEPTIC ARTHRITIS

In various series, elbow involvement ranges from 6% to 12% in patients with septic joints.[5, 8, 10] Risk is increased in patients with rheumatoid arthritis.[11] As with infection of other joints, the key to diagnosis is joint aspiration. *Staphylococcus* is the usual pathogen in adults.[6, 8, 10, 15]

Drainage of the joint is essential. This may be accomplished through serial aspiration or surgery. Controversy exists as to use of initial conservative or surgical management of septic arthritis. Arthroscopic debridement of the knee for septic arthritis is a well-established treatment option. Elbow arthroscopy for an infected elbow involving irrigation, debridement of loculations and adhesions, and partial synovectomy and placement of drains, is also worthwhile.[13, 20]

Arthroscopy may also be useful if the diagnosis of septic arthritis is uncertain. Arthroscopically assisted synovial biopsy may also allow establishment of the diagnosis.

Technique. The surgeon should perform standard diagnostic arthroscopy of all compartments of the elbow. Copious irrigation in each compartment should be performed

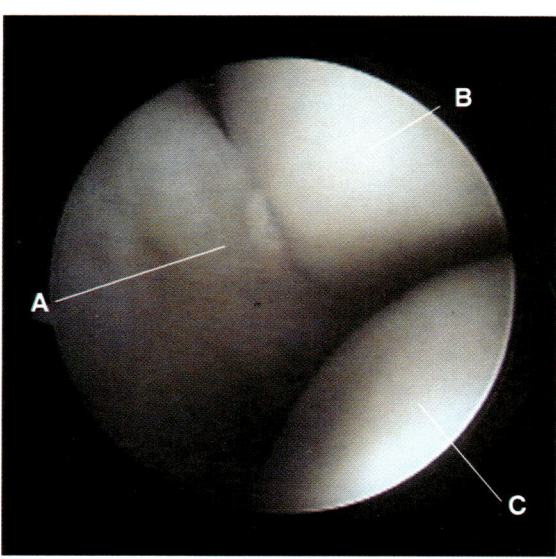

FIG 6–20. View obtained with the arthroscope in the lateral compartment. A plica *(a)* impinges on the radial head *(b)* as it articulates with the capitellum. *c*, the plica can be removed through the accessory lateral portal, with subsequent resolution of symptoms.

through large bore inflow and outflow cannulas. Loculations and adhesions should be debrided with the shaver. Partial synovectomy of inflamed synovium may be helpful (see p. 87–88). Closed suction drainage tubes are placed anteriorly and posteriorly after arthroscopy is completed.

TREATMENT OF ELBOW FRACTURES

Arthroscopy may be helpful in the management of fractures of the radial head, capitellum, or olecranon.[2, 7, 14, 22] Excision of chondral or osteochondral fracture fragments and evaluation of fracture displacement are indications for arthroscopy. Percutaneous pinning or other forms of reduction and internal fixation with arthroscopic assistance is useful only in very select cases.[7, 14, 16, 22] More commonly, fracture fragments blocking elbow motion are removed. Hemarthrosis from acute fractures may lead to early termination of arthroscopy because of poor visualization.

Technique. Excision of chondral or osteochondral fragments has been described (see Chapter 5), but there are some additional technical tips with regard to fractures. In acute fracture dislocations of the elbow, one should not attempt arthroscopy because of the risk of fluid extravasation and subsequent neurovascular injury. In a patient with an acute fracture only, anterolateral and anteromedial portals should be established in the standard fashion. The shaver should be used through one portal to remove the hemarthrosis and debris. An additional outflow cannula several centimeters proximal to the anteromedial portal may help improve visualization. Removal of a large fracture fragment in one piece requires a significant increase in the size of the capsular portal and skin with a knife. This often causes fluid extravasation through the large capsular hole into the soft tissues, and may lead to neurovascular injury. To avoid this, large fracture fragments should be removed in small pieces through the original portal.

Case 4: Elbow Fracture

A 42-year-old woman who sustained a fall 8 months previously complains of left elbow stiffness. Range of motion is from 20 to 110 degrees of flexion (Figs 6–21-6–25).

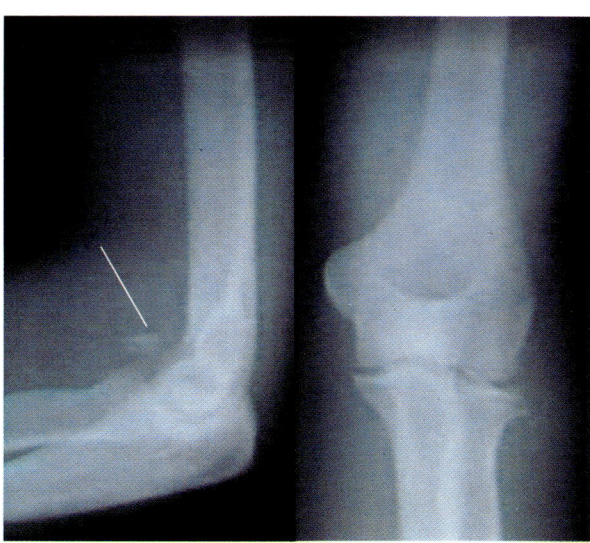

FIG 6–21. Lateral and anteroposterior radiographs reveal a fracture fragment from the radial head lodged in the anterior compartment.

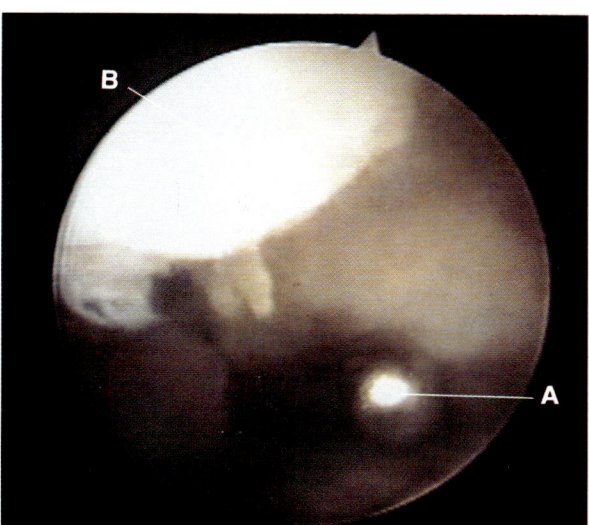

FIG 6–22. The arthroscope is in the anterolateral portal, and a shaver (a) is in the anteromedial portal. Adhesions have been debrided. A fracture fragment (b) is adherent to the anterior capsule.

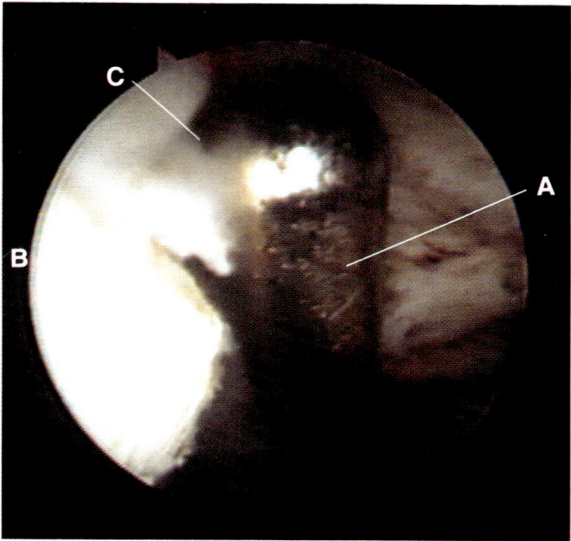

FIG 6–23. A shaver (a) is used to debride around the fracture fragment (b) to free it from the anterior capsule (c).

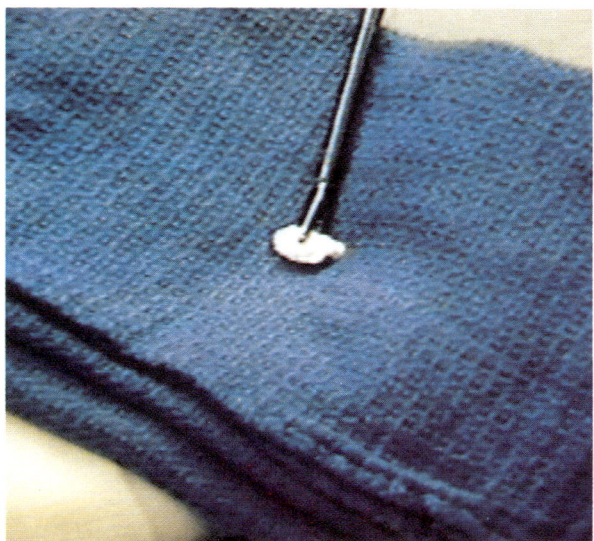

FIG 6–24. The fracture fragment has been removed with a grasper.

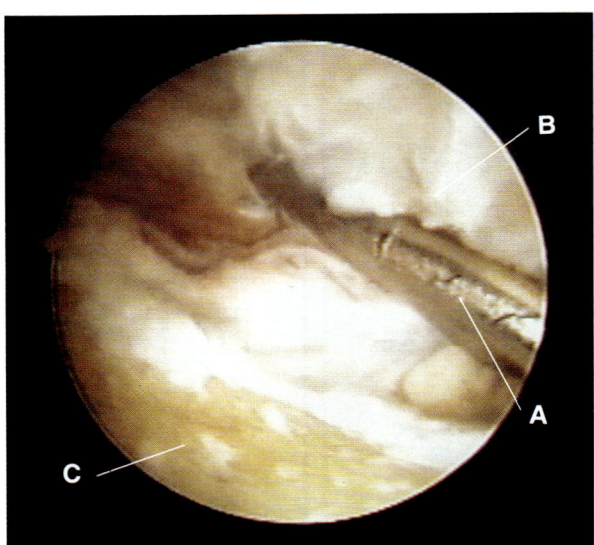

FIG 6-25. A shaver *(a)* is used to remove remaining adhesions *(b)* from the anterior compartment. *c,* anterior humerus.

REFERENCES

1. Amis AA, Hughes SJ, Miller JH, et al: A functional study of the rheumatoid elbow, *Rheumatol Rehab* 21:151, 1982.
2. Andrews JR, Carson WG: Arthroscopy of the elbow, Arthroscopy 1:97, 1985.
3. Clarke RP: Symptomatic, lateral synovial fringe (plica) of the elbow joint, *Arthroscopy* 4:112, 1988.
4. Commandre FA, Taillan B, Benezis C, et al: Plicae synovialis (synovial fold) of the elbow, *J Sports Med Phys Fitness* 28:209, 1988.
5. Goldenberg DO, Brandt KD, Cohen AS, et al: Treatment of septic arthritis: comparison of knee aspiration and surgery as initial modes of joint drainage, *Arthr Rheum* 18:83, 1975.
6. Goldenberg DO, Reed JI: Bacterial arthritis, *N Engl J Med* 312:764, 1985.
7. Guhl JF: Arthroscopy and arthroscopic surgery of the elbow, *Orthopaedics* 8:290, 1985.
8. Jackson MA, Nelson JD: Etiology and medical management of acute bone and joint infections and pediatric patients, *J Pediatr Orthop* 2:313, 1982.
9. Jeffries TE: Synovial chondromatosis, *J Bone Joint Surg [Br]* 49:530, 1967.
10. Kelley PJ, Martin WJ, Coventry MB: Bacterial (suppurative) arthritis in the adult, *J Bone Joint Surg [Am]* 52:1595, 1970.
11. Kellgren JH, Ball J, Fairbrother RW, et al: Suppurative arthritis complicating rheumatoid arthritis, *Br Med J* 1:1193, 1958.
12. Milgram JW: Synovial osteochondromatosis, *J Bone Joint Surg [Am]* 59:792, 1977.
13. Morrey BF: *The elbow and its disorders,* Philadelphia, 1985, Saunders.
14. O'Driscoll SW, Morrey BF: Arthroscopy of the elbow: diagnostic and therapeutic benefits and hazards, *J Bone Joint Surg [Am]* 74:84, 1992.
15. O'Meara PM, Bartal E: Septic arthritis: process, etiology, treatment, outcome, *Orthopaedics* 11:623, 1988.
16. Poehling GG, Whipple TL, Sisco L, et al: Elbow arthroscopy: a new technique, *Arthroscopy* 5:222, 1989.
17. Porter BB, Richardson C, Vainio K: Rheumatoid arthritis of the elbow: the results of synovectomy, *J Bone Joint Surg [Br]* 56:427, 1974.
18. Raunio P: Synovectomy of the elbow in rheumatoid arthritis, *Reconstr Surg Traumatol* 18:63, 1981.
19. Sakkers RJB, DeJong D, Van der Heul KO: X-chromosome inactivation in patients who have pigmented villonodular synovitis, *J Bone Joint Surg [Am]* 73:1532, 1991.
20. Sheppard JE, Marion JD, Hurst DI: Arthroscopic elbow surgery: five-year experience and observations in forty-eight cases, *Am J Arthroscopy* 1:13, 1991.
21. Spjut HJ, Dorfman HD, Fechner RE, et al: *Tumors of bone and cartilage,* Washington, DC, Armed Forces Institute of Pathology, 1983.
22. Woods GW: Elbow arthroscopy, *Clin Sports Med* 6:557, 1987.

Chapter 7

Complications of Elbow Arthroscopy

William G. Carson, Jr., M.D.

As with any surgical procedure, complications may occur from elbow arthroscopy. Complications are usually associated with inexperience, poor technique, and unfamiliarity with superficial and arthroscopic anatomy. One goal of this textbook is to increase the fund of knowledge of elbow arthroscopic anatomy, pathologic conditions, and surgical techniques so that potential complications may be avoided.

TYPES OF COMPLICATIONS

Complications of elbow arthroscopy are similar to those encountered with any arthroscopic procedure and include infection, problems associated with the use of a tourniquet, instrument breakage, iatrogenic scuffing of articular surfaces, and neurovascular complications.[3,5,8] Infection is infrequent with elbow arthroscopy because of the large amount of fluid passed through the joint during the surgical procedure and the small incisions required for the arthroscopic instrumentation. The causes of neurovascular complications and their prevention are the focus of this chapter.

NEUROVASCULAR COMPLICATIONS

Neurovascular complications, appear to be more of a problem than infection. Neurovascular structures at risk during arthroscopy of the elbow include the radial nerve, median nerve, brachial artery ulnar nerve, and the many subcutaneous nerves about the elbow.

During initiation of the anterolateral arthroscopic portal, structures at risk include the posterior antebrachial cutaneous nerve, the lateral antebrachial cutaneous nerve, and the radial nerve (Fig 7–1). In establishment of the anteromedial portal, structures at risk include the medial antebrachial cutaneous nerve, the median nerve, and the brachial artery (Fig 7–2). Structures at risk during establishment of the posterolateral portal include the lateral brachial cutaneous nerve and the posterior antebrachial cutaneous nerve (Fig 7–3). Structures at risk in establishment of the accessory arthroscopic portals, such as the "soft spot" or direct lateral portal, include the posterior antebrachial cutaneous nerve. With establishment of the accessory straight or transtriceps arthroscopic portal, structures at risk include the posterior antebrachial cutaneous nerve and the ulnar nerve.

Multiple complications related to arthroscopy of the elbow have been reported, and

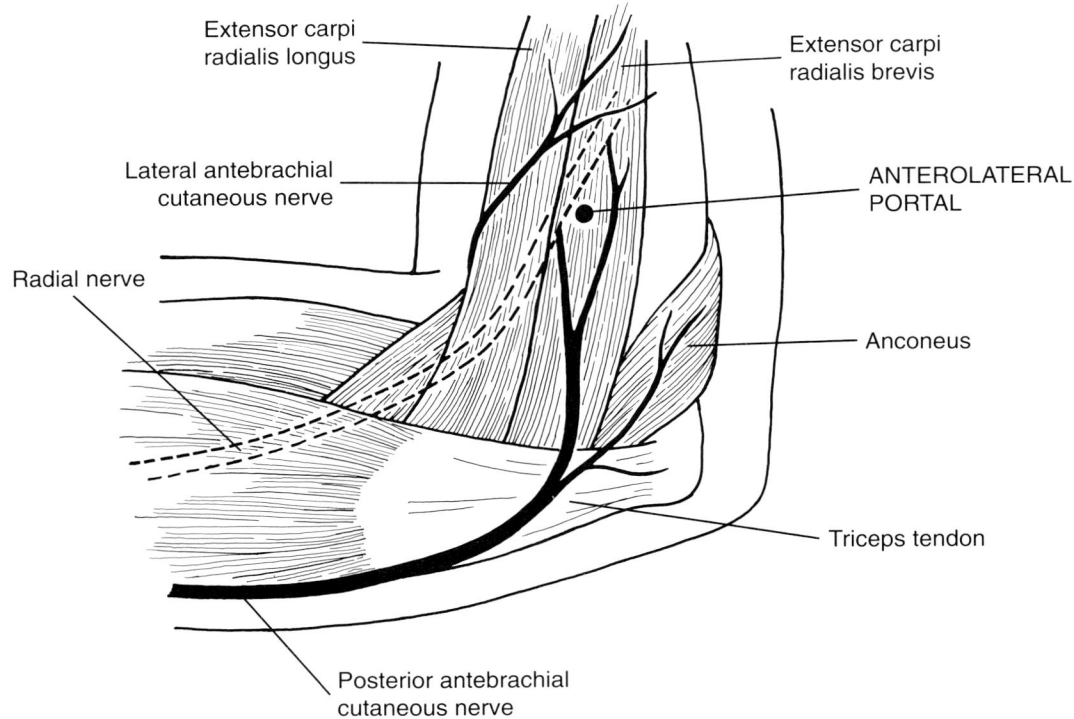

FIG 7–1. Portal anatomy of anterolateral portal. (Modified from Lynch GJ, et al: Neurovascular anatomy of elbow arthroscopy: inherent risks, *Arthroscopy* 2:192, 1986.)

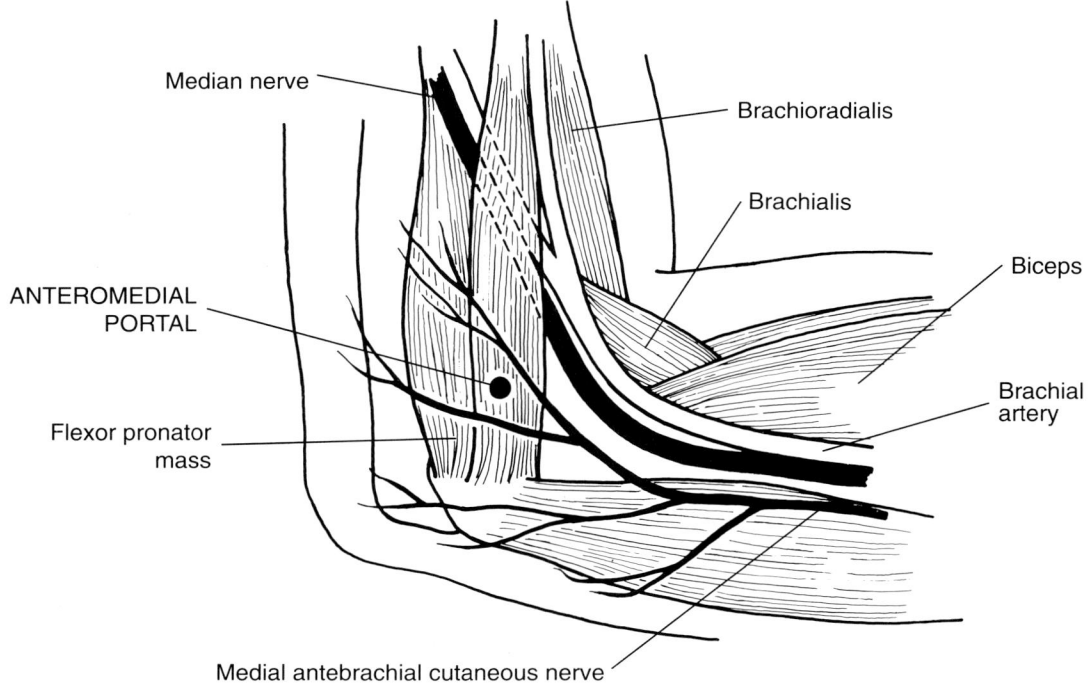

FIG 7–2. Portal anatomy of anteromedial portal. (Modified from Lynch GJ, et al: Neurovascular anatomy of elbow arthroscopy: inherent risks, *Arthroscopy* 2:192, 1986.)

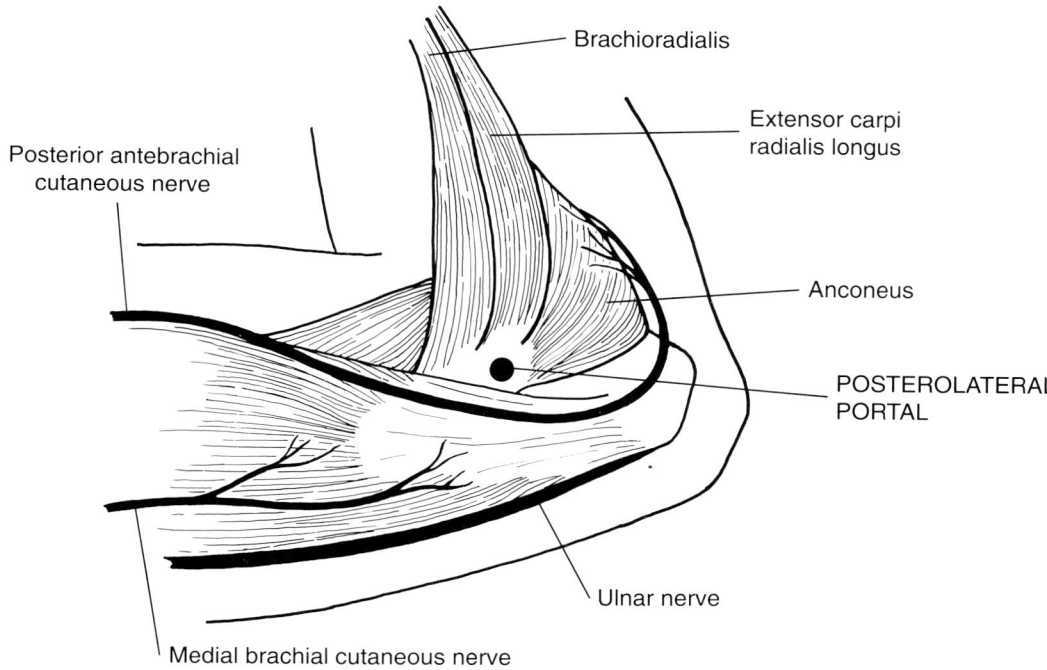

FIG 7–3. Portal anatomy of posterolateral portal. (Modified from Lynch GJ, et al: Neurovascular anatomy of elbow arthroscopy: inherent risks, *Arthroscopy* 2:192, 1986.)

most of these relate to neurovascular complications. In a series of 21 elbow arthroscopies, Lynch et al.[11] reported one transient low radial nerve palsy, a transient low median nerve palsy, and formation of a neuroma of the medial antebrachial cutaneous nerve. It was believed that the transient low radial nerve palsy was the result of overdistention of the joint, and the condition resolved in 8 hours. The transient low median nerve palsy was believed to be secondary to use of a local anesthetic. The neuroma of the medial antebrachial cutaneous nerve ultimately required resection.

Casscells[7] described a case of irreparable damage to the ulnar nerve during abrasion arthroplasty of the elbow. Thomas et al.[17] described a radial nerve injury, and Papilion[14] described compression neuropathy of the radial nerve during elbow arthroscopy. In a series of 45 patients, Guhl[9] reported one injury to the sensory branch of the radial nerve, and Morrey[12] reported a transient radial nerve palsy secondary to fluid extravasation. In a series of 24 arthroscopies reported by Andrews and Carson, one patient experienced a transient median nerve palsy. This transient nerve palsy was believed to be secondary to leakage of local anesthetic from the capsule, causing a temporary nerve block. Since the writing of this textbook in 1992, the senior editor (JRA) has encountered one case of transient ulnar neuropraxia occurring after posteromedial osteophyte removal.

In a survey of members of the Arthroscopy Association of North America, 395,556 surgical arthroscopic procedures were evaluated; 569 of these were elbow arthroscopies. The respondents were performing on average 0.74 elbow arthroscopies per month, and had been performing surgical elbow arthroscopy on average 3.9 years. Of this entire group, only one reported a neurovascular complication, a radial nerve injury.[16] I am also aware of undocumented cases of compartment syndrome of the forearm, complete transection of the median nerve, and complete transection of the radial nerve secondary to elbow arthroscopy.

Thus, injuries to the subcutaneous or deeper nerves about the elbow have been reported, with the injuries occurring either secondary to actual surgical transection or possibly from fluid extravasation during the surgical procedure or the use of a tourniquet. The other consideration is traction or blunt trauma to the various nerves about the elbow. Injury to the brachial artery has not been reported; it appears to be somewhat protected because it lies directly toward the middle of the joint and is lateral to the median nerve when the medial portal is established, and medial to the radial nerve when the lateral portal is established. It appears that the radial nerve is most at risk in performance of elbow arthroscopy.

INITIAL ARTHROSCOPIC PORTAL: MEDIAL VS. LATERAL

The anterolateral portal has usually been described as the portal to be established first in performance of arthroscopy of the elbow.[1, 4, 6] This anterolateral portal enters the elbow just anterior to the radial head. The anterolateral portal has commonly been initiated with the patient in the supine position. Much recent interest, however, has been shown in use of the prone approach in combination with a proximal medial[2, 15] or medial[10] arthroscopic portal as the initial arthroscopic portal to be established. Poehling[15] and Lindenfeld[10] and others who advocate a medial approach as the initial arthroscopic approach have demonstrated that the distance between the median nerve and the medial arthroscopic instruments is increased compared with minimal distance between the lateral arthroscopic instruments and the radial nerve in establishment of these lateral portals. Lindenfeld[10] inserted polyurethane foam to distend the elbow capsule in six cadaver specimens. The foam was allowed to harden, and the specimens were dissected with the medial and lateral portals established, and the proximity of the neurovascular structures to the portals was established. It was found that the anterolateral portal that was established 3 cm distal and 1 cm anterior to the lateral humeral epicondyle extended on average to within 2.8 mm of the radial nerve. The medial portal (1 cm proximal and 1 cm anterior to the medial humeral epicondyle), however, extended on average to within 22 mm to the median nerve. The ulnar nerve was 25 mm from the medial portal.

Verhaan et al[18] performed cadaveric dissections of five specimens with plastic rods in place through the anteromedial and anterolateral portals. These dissections were performed without elbow distention, and it was seen that in establishment of the anterolateral portal, the radial nerve was on average 17 mm from the entering instruments, and the deep branch of the radial nerve 7 mm away. In establishment of the anteromedial portal the median nerve was on average 18 mm from the arthroscopic instruments, the brachial artery 26 mm away, and the ulnar nerve always at least 26 mm away. Lynch et al.[11] performed dissections of nondistended and distended elbows and found that in the anterolateral portal the radial nerve was on average 4 mm away when the elbow was nondistended, but this distance increased to 11 mm with elbow distention. In establishment of the anteromedial portal, they found that the median nerve was 3 to 10 mm from the instruments; this increased, however, to 14 mm with distention. Andrews and Carson[1], in dissections of nondistended elbows, found that the radial nerve was approximately 7 mm from the arthroscopic instruments in the anterolateral portal and that the median nerve was approximately 10 mm from the arthroscopic instruments in establishment of the anteromedial portal. Therefore, with regard to nerve injury, it appears from these cadaveric dissections that the margin of safety appears to be greater during establishment of the medial portals than during establishment of the anterolateral portals. Advocates of the proximal medial portals believe there is less risk to neurovascular structures, not only because there is greater distance between the instruments and the neurovascular structures but also because the instruments enter parallel to the neurovascular structures as they progress toward the elbow joint, causing less chance of injury. With the standard anteromedial or anterolateral portals, the entering instruments approach at an angle from

60 to 90 degrees to the neurovascular structures, and in theory would appear to place these structures at more risk. The senior editor (JRA) continues to establish the anteromedial portal under direct visualization from the anterolateral portal (see Chapter 4), and has found this to be an extremely safe and reliable technique.

PREVENTION OF COMPLICATIONS

Most of the complications of elbow arthroscopy can be prevented by adhering to a strict surgical technique, with attention to detail and acute awareness of the portal and neurovascular anatomy of the elbow. Three of the most important aspects of elbow arthroscopy are simple measures, such as the use of a skin marker to mark the bony anatomy before initiation of the surgery and the use of an 18-gauge spinal needle as a precursor to larger arthroscopic instruments (Fig 7-4). The principle of having the elbow joint maximally distended at all times to further displace the neurovascular structures away from the entering arthroscopic instruments is also important. Lynch et al.[11] demonstrated that when 35 to 40 mL of fluid is inserted into the elbow, the radial nerve moves an additional 7 mm anterior and away from the entering arthroscopic instruments. Also, the elbow should be kept at 90 degrees of flexion throughout the majority of the arthroscopic procedure, to further relax the neurovascular structures in the antecubital fossa.

The surgeon should be aware not only of the deeper neurovascular structures, such as the radial nerve and median nerve, but of the presence of the many cutaneous nerves about the elbow. A small incision should be made into the skin, not a "stab incision" as is often used in the shoulder or the knee, and a No. 11 blade should simply be laid across the skin, and the skin then pulled across the blade. This incision may then be deepened through underlying subcutaneous tissues with the use of a hemostat. A blunt rather than a sharp trocar is used because it can be readily inserted through the subcutaneous fat and musculotendinous structures and thereby minimize damage to nearby neurovascular structures and the articular cartilage.

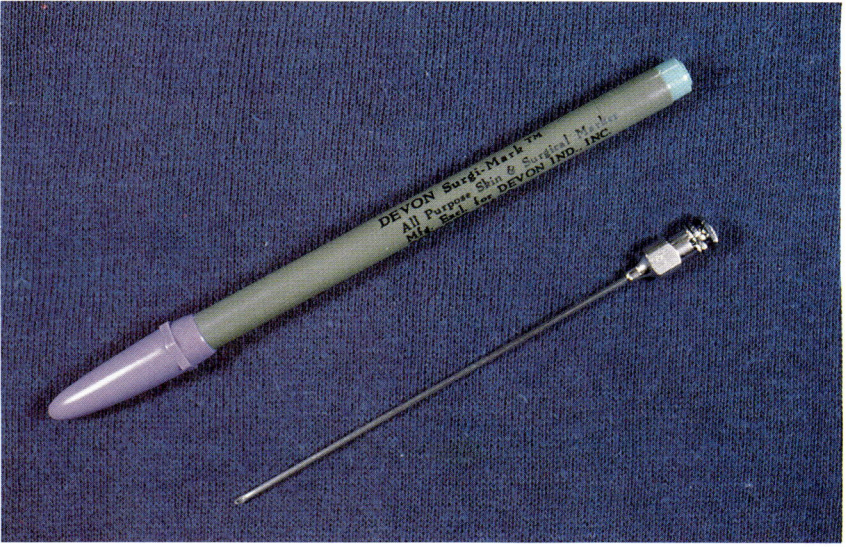

FIG 7-4. Essential items for safe elbow arthroscopy include an 18-gauge spinal needle and a skin marker.

Fluid extravasation during arthroscopy of the elbow can create technical difficulties as well as risks to both deep and subcutaneous neurovascular structures. Lynch et al.[11] and O'Driscoll et al.[13] measured the intraarticular pressure of the elbow in 13 fresh frozen human cadaver specimens. The capacity of the elbow joint capsule was approximately 23 mL ± 4 mL. The intraarticular pressure was the lowest at 80 degrees of flexion, and capsular rupture occurred at relatively low intraarticular pressures. Arthroscopy of the elbow should be performed slowly and deliberately, to avoid having the arthroscope slip out of the capsule or the inflow cannulas slip back and thereby cause increased leakage of fluid and further technical difficulties. Because fluid extravasates extracapsularly in the subcutaneous tissues, this could further compress the capsule, making reentry of the elbow joint increasingly difficult (Fig 7–5).

Proper cannulas should be used. These should have openings at the end of the cannula only, and no "side vents" (Fig 7–6), because if side-vented cannulas slip back during the arthroscopic procedure the fluid could be placed in the subcutaneous tissues rather than in the joint itself. Use of an interchangeable cannula system avoids multiple passes through the capsule and thus helps minimize extravasation. When proceeding from compartment to compartment during arthroscopy, we have found it helpful to leave cannulas in place in the previous compartment; then if it is necessary to return to a previous compartment, access is easily obtained through these cannulas, and repuncture of these compartments is avoided.

Another principle for minimization of fluid extravasation in arthroscopy of the elbow is to use motorized instruments when possible. Handheld instruments often require multiple passes in and out of the elbow joint, causing risks for further capsular holes and further fluid extravasation. Rubber gasket–type disposable cannulas are available that can help limit fluid extravasation by sealing off the arthroscopic portal as the instruments are being used (Fig 7–7).

Complications of elbow arthroscopy can also be avoided with proper patient selection and by use of proper indications. The main indication for arthroscopy of the elbow is loose body removal. The use of arthroscopy for treatment of bony ankylosis or severe fibrous ankylosis is contraindicated because arthroscopic instruments are difficult to insert

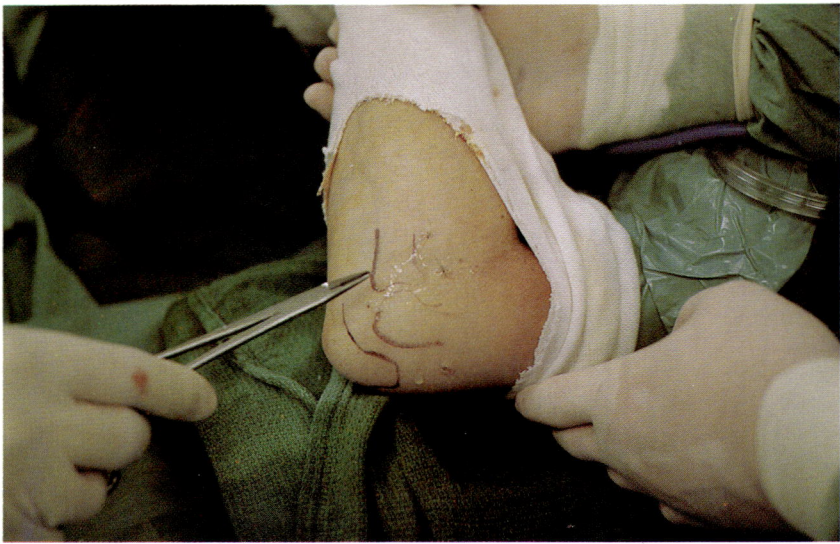

FIG 7–5. Example of postoperative fluid extravasation after elbow arthroscopy.

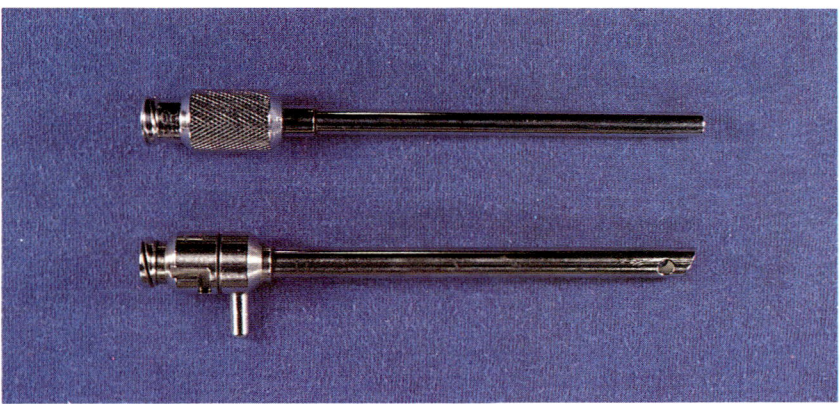

FIG 7–6. Example of correct (nonvented) inflow cannula and incorrect (vented) inflow cannula.

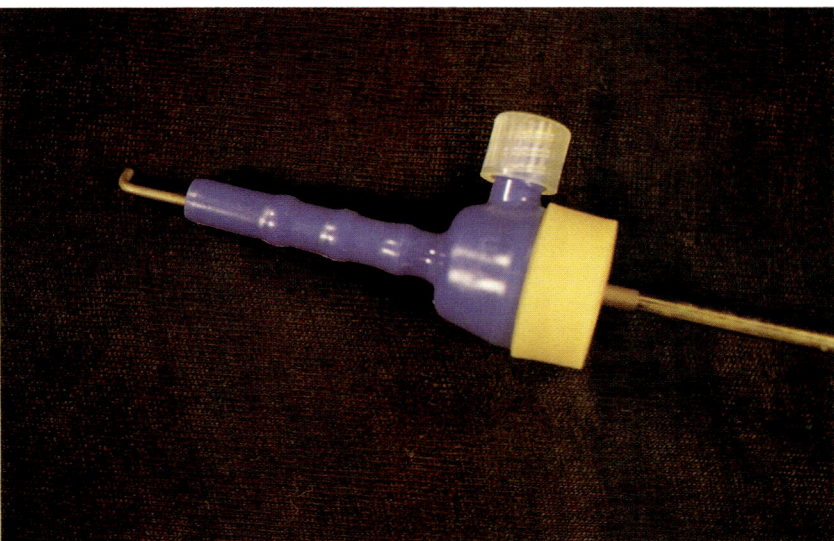

FIG 7–7. Example of disposable rubber-seal cannula for minimization of fluid extravasation (Acufex Universal Cannula; Acufex Microsurgical, Norwood, Mass.)

into the elbow, and repeated attempts to insert instruments into the elbow in a contracted capsular space could lead to neurovascular damage, articular cartilage scuffing, and substantial extracapsular fluid extravasation. Surgical procedures such as anterior transposition of the ulnar nerve or other procedures that have altered the anatomy about the elbow such that neurovascular structures are in jeopardy may also be contraindications for elbow arthroscopy.

CONCLUSIONS

Arthroscopy of the elbow is a technically demanding surgical procedure, and considerable attention to detail is essential for a safe and reproducible arthroscopic examination to be performed. Complications can be avoided by adhering to a strict surgical technique.

REFERENCES

1. Andrews JR, Carson WG: Arthroscopy of the elbow, *Arthroscopy* 1:97–107, 1985.
2. Baker CL, Shalvoy RM: The prone position for elbow arthroscopy, *Clin Sports Med* 10:623–628, 1991.
3. Burman MS: Arthroscopy or the direct visualization of joints, *J Bone Joint Surg* 13:669–695, 1931.
4. Carson WG: Arthroscopy of the elbow, *Instr Course Lect* 37:195–201, 1988.
5. Carson WG: Complications of elbow arthroscopy. In Minkoff J, Sherman O, editors: *Arthroscopic surgery,* Baltimore, 1988, Williams & Wilkins, pp 166–179.
6. Carson WG, Meyer JF: Diagnostic arthroscopy of the elbow: surgical technique and arthroscopic and portal anatomy. In McGinty JB, editor: *Operative arthroscopy,* New York, 1991, Raven Press, p 584.
7. Casscells SW: Neurovascular anatomy and elbow arthroscopy: inherent risks (editor's comment), *Arthroscopy* 2:190, 1987.
8. DeLee JC: Complications of arthroscopy and arthroscopic surgery: results of a national survey, *Arthroscopy* 1:214–220, 1985.
9. Guhl JF: Arthroscopy and arthroscopic surgery of the elbow, *Orthopedics* 8:290–296, 1985.
10. Lindenfeld TN: Medial approach in elbow arthroscopy, *Am J Sports Med* 18:413–417, 1990.
11. Lynch GJ, Meyers JF, Whipple TL, et al: Neurovascular anatomy and elbow arthroscopy: inherent risks, *Arthroscopy* 2:191–197, 1986.
12. Morrey BF: Arthroscopy of the elbow, *Inst Course Lect* 35:102, 1986.
13. O'Driscoll SW, Morrey BF, An K: Intra-articular pressure and capacity of the elbow, *Arthroscopy* 6:100–103, 1990.
14. Papilion JD, Neff RS, Shall LM: Compression neuropathy of the radial nerve as a complication of elbow arthroscopy: a case report and review of the literature, *Arthroscopy* 4:284–286, 1988.
15. Poehling GG, Whipple TL, Sisco L, et al: Elbow arthroscopy: a new technique, *Arthroscopy* 5:222–224, 1989.
16. Small NC: Complications in arthroscopy: on knee and other joints, *Arthroscopy* 2:253–258, 1986.
17. Thomas MA, Fast A, Shapiro D: Radial nerve damage as a complication of an elbow arthroscopy, *Clin Orthop* 215:130–131, 1987.
18. Verhaan J, VanMameren H, Brandsma A: Risks of neurovascular injury in elbow arthroscopy: starting anteromedially or anterolaterally?, *Arthroscopy* 7:287–290, 1991.

Chapter 8

Rehabilitation of the Elbow Following Arthroscopic Surgery

Kevin E. Wilk, PT

As indications for elbow arthroscopy expand and arthroscopic equipment and techniques improve, performance of arthroscopy will increase. It is therefore imperative for both orthopedists and physical therapists to become knowledgeable in postoperative rehabilitation techniques to help guide patients along the road to full recovery.

Rehabilitation following elbow surgery is relatively common in orthopedic and sports physical therapy practices; however, relatively little regarding the rehabilitation process following elbow surgery has been written.[20,26] The unique anatomic orientation of the elbow complex, consisting of three bones articulating to form four articulations, contributes to a high degree of joint congruence and accounts for much of the difficulty experienced by the therapist in obtaining normal function following an elbow injury or surgery. Because of the many unique anatomic considerations, as previously discussed in this book, the therapist is faced with multiple clinical challenges to rehabilitate the injured elbow successfully.[32] With the advent of improved surgical techniques and the arthroscope, the frequently experienced postsurgery complications such as loss of motion,[1,4,11] loss of muscle and strength,[12] and paresthesia have been minimized.[3] The purpose of this chapter is to discuss these clinical enigmas and suggest possible treatment options that may lead to a successful outcome following arthroscopic elbow surgery.

Rehabilitation after an elbow injury or elbow surgery follows a multiphased course that is sequential and progressive. The ultimate goal of this process is return of the patient or athlete to activity as quickly and safely as possible. To enable the athlete to return to sports activities or strenuous work, the elbow must exhibit (1) full, nonpainful range of motion, (2) no pain or tenderness at clinical examination, (3) satisfactory muscular strength, power, and endurance, and (4) a satisfactory clinical examination. Once these criteria have been met, the patient may gradually return to sports activities in a controlled, progressive manner.

BASIC PRINCIPLES

Briefly, there are six basic principles for any rehabilitation program:

1. Effects of immobilization must be minimized.
2. Healing tissue must never be overstressed.

3. Patient must fulfill specific criteria to progress from phase to phase.
4. Rehabilitation program must be based on current clinical and scientific research.
5. Program must be adaptable to the specific goals of each patient.
6. Rehabilitation program must be a team effort, with the orthopaedist, therapist, trainer, and patient all working together.

These basic treatment principles are followed throughout the rehabilitation process for both surgical and nonsurgical elbow conditions. The rehabilitation process is a team approach, with all members working together toward the common goal of returning the patient to unrestricted competition as quickly and safely as possible. The members of the rehabilitation team include the patient, physician, therapist, athletic trainer, coach, and biomechanist, and in many cases, the team is expanded to include the family of the athlete. The key to successful rehabilitation of any athlete is communication between the team members. This communication is essential to ensure appropriate progression and expectations in every phase of the rehabilitation program. Patient education by each team member during each phase in the rehabilitative process will improve compliance which should improve the chances of successful rehabilitation.

REHABILITATION

Phase 1

In the first phase of elbow rehabilitation, the immediate motion phase, the goals are to (1) reestablish nonpainful range of motion, (2) decrease pain and inflammation, and (3) retard muscular atrophy. The exercise prescription must be designed to minimize the effects of immobilization in both surgical and nonsurgical instances and to respect the healing constraints of the tissues involved.

Early range of motion exercises are performed to nourish the articular cartilage and assist in collagen tissue synthesis and organization.[21-24, 28] Active assisted and passive range of motion exercises in all planes of elbow and wrist motion are used to prevent deleterious scar formation and adhesion development. A major advantage of arthroscopic elbow surgery is its minimal mobilizing of tissue, allowing immediate motion to be performed following most procedures. Reestablishment of full elbow extension is a primary goal in this initial phase of rehabilitation. A common side effect when this goal is not successfully accomplished is an elbow flexion contracture.[1, 11, 20] When this occurs in a throwing patient, abnormal stresses are placed on various elbow structures.[2] These repetitive abnormal stresses may lead to microtraumatic or macrotraumatic injury.[2]

Many factors predispose patients to an elbow flexion contracture, including (1) intimate congruency of the elbow complex, especially of the humeroulnar joint; (2) tightness of the elbow capsule; and (3) tendency of the anterior capsule to scar and become adhesive. The anterior capsule is relatively thin, and is very sensitive to injury. This may lead to many alterations in its anatomy, which adversely affect the normal motion. The medial and lateral ligamentous structures are subject to rupture, contracture, and occasionally calcification, which can severely compromise normal motion. Posttraumatic thickening of the lateral ligamentous structures can often cause impingement and snapping during elbow movements.[20] Also, the anterior anatomy of the elbow is unique in that the brachialis muscle inserts into capsule and crosses the anterior aspect as a muscle and not as a tendinous tissue. Injury to the elbow may lead to the formation of excessive scar tissue by the brachialis muscle and may also cause functional splinting of the elbow. Once motion is limited, changes can occur to the sarcomere of the muscle, which will lead to an additional loss in motion.[10, 27, 34]

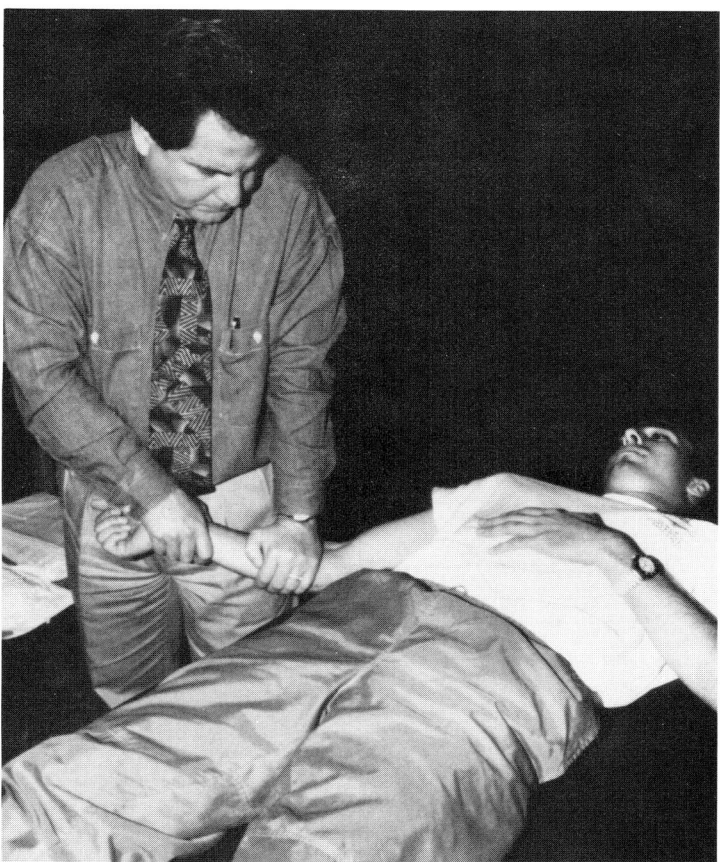

FIG 8–1. Joint mobilization technique to increase elbow extension. This technique utilizes a posterior glide of the ulna on the distal humerus.

To counteract these capsular restrictions, joint mobilization is performed to both the humeroulnar and humeroradial joints.[14, 17] To regain elbow extension, a posterior glide of the ulna on the humerus is performed (Fig 8–1).[14] During this phase, grade 3 mobilizations are performed to produce a slight stretch on the anterior capsule (Table 8–1); in later phases of the rehabilitation program grade 4 mobilizations are performed to produce a greater stretch on the capsule.[17] This type of aggressive mobilization is not performed until pain has been eliminated. Another extremely effective exercise designed to obtain

TABLE 8–1.

Joint Mobilization Grades of Oscillation*

Grade	Description
1	Small amplitude glides performed in the beginning portion of motion, to neuromodulate pain and improve joint lubrication; minimal stretch on capsule
2	Large amplitude glides performed in the middle range of motion, to neuromodulate pain and improve joint lubrication; moderate stress to the capsule
3	Large amplitude glides performed in the middle range to end range, to stretch the capsule; moderate stress
4	Small amplitude glides performed in the end range, to produce pronounced stretch on capsule and ligaments

*Modified from Maitland GD: *Vertebral manipulation,* London, 1977, Butterworth.

full elbow extension is passive elbow extension with a handheld weight, to produce a passive overpressure extension stretch (Fig 8–2). A fulcrum (e.g., a towel roll) is placed posterior to the elbow joint to effect greater extension moment during this activity. This stretch is performed for 2 to 3 minutes, with a low weight, for a low-intensity stretch of long duration. In the literature, this low–intensity, long-duration stretch has been reported to induce a plastic response of the collagen tissue that will result in permanent elongation of the collagen tissues.[15, 25, 29, 30] This exercise is extremely beneficial for achievement of full elbow extension with programs followed at home. We recommend that this passive elbow extension stretch be performed three to four times per day at home, to contradict the early signs of a flexion contracture.

A second goal in this phase is to decrease pain and inflammation. Grade I and II joint mobilization techniques are used to neuromodulate pain by stimulating the type I and II articular receptors of the joint.[17] These joint mobilization techniques are small oscillations designed to cause minimal to moderate amounts of joint distraction and are performed in the beginning to middle range of capsular motion. They should assist in pain relief.[17] Other modalities are used to diminish pain and inflammation, such as ice, high-voltage pulsed galvanic stimulation, and transcutaneous neuromuscular stimulation as required. Ultrasound or a warm whirlpool bath can be used at the onset of treatment to prepare the tissue for stretching and assist in improving the extensibility of the capsule and musculotendinous unit once the acute inflammatory and effused phase has passed. It has been suggested that a higher ultrasound frequency be used if this modality is chosen; this will result in greater attenuation and absorption of energy in the structures such as the anterior capsule of the elbow. Because the capsule is 1 to 2 cm below the skin surface, a frequency of 3 mHz is recommended.[35]

During this phase, additional focus is placed on retardation of the muscular atrophy of the elbow and wrist musculature. Patients are instructed to perform submaximal iso-

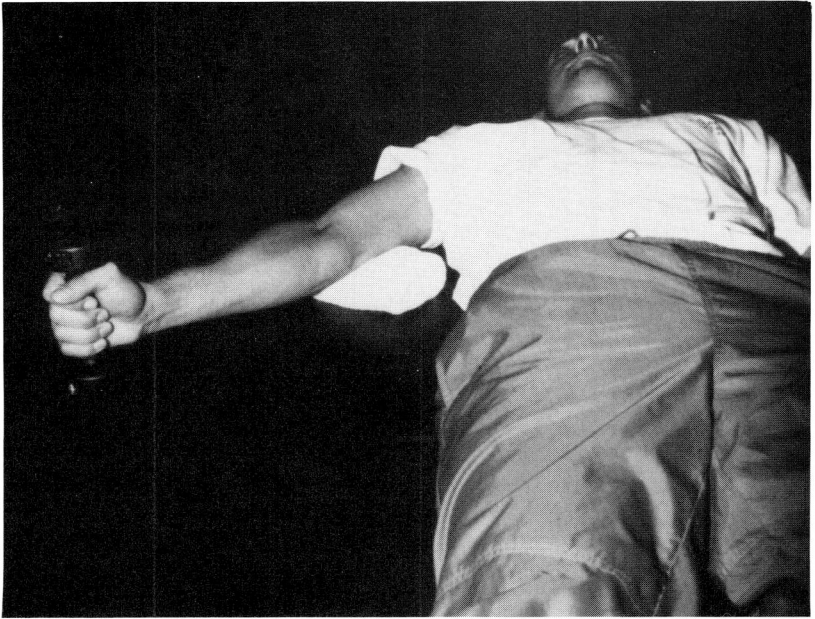

FIG 8–2. Passive elbow extension stretch with handheld weight to cause overpressure into extension. This stretch is performed for long duration with low resistance. The towel roll creates a fulcrum for the stretch.

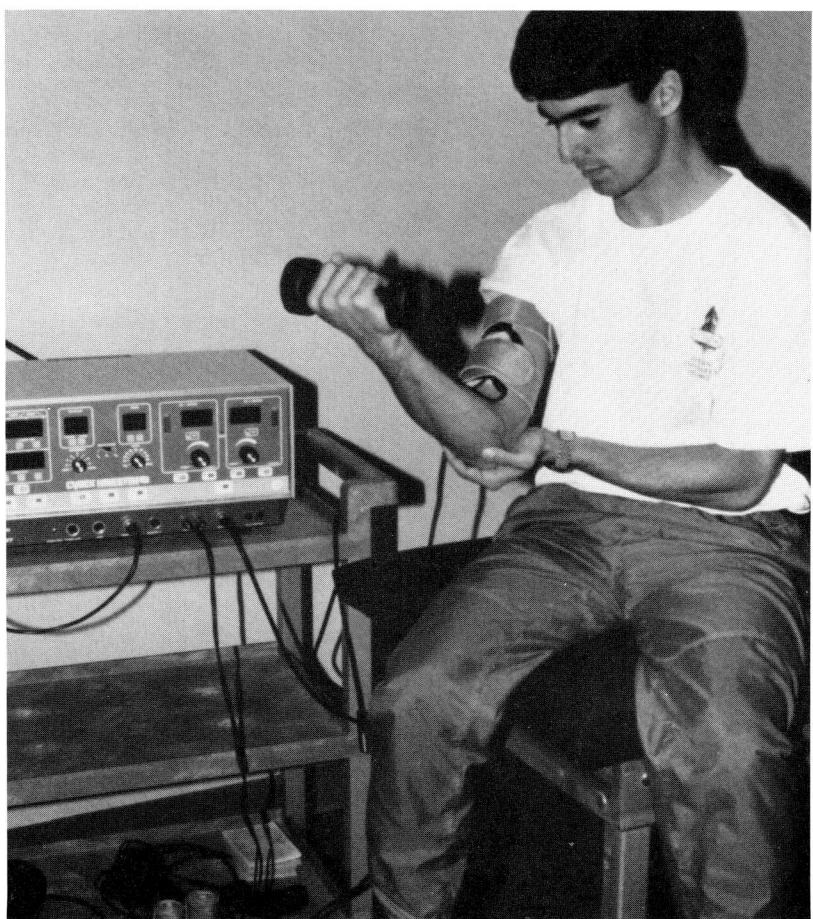

FIG 8–3. Electrical muscle stimulation is applied to the biceps brachii muscle to enhance the active resisted contraction and to assist in muscular hypertrophy.

metric exercises for the elbow flexors and extensors and the wrist flexor, extensor, pronator, and supinator muscle groups. These isometric exercises are performed at multiple angles for three to five sets of 10 repetitions, with each contraction held for 6 to 8 seconds. Electrical muscle stimulation to augment voluntary muscular contraction may assist in retardation of muscular atrophy (Fig 8–3).[1, 7, 9, 16, 18] These muscle groups are emphasized because of the substantial role they have during sport activities.[8, 13]

In this first phase of elbow rehabilitation the primary goal is to obtain full elbow extension. By reaching this goal, the organization and alignment of collagen fibers is improved, and the most common side effect, elbow flexion contracture, is prevented. Stretching must be performed with caution to ensure that the healing tissues are not overstressed or that the patient's pain complaints are not substantially increased.[19] The pain-resistance sequence is evaluated in conjunction with the range of motion end feels to determine how aggressive a stretching program should be (Table 8–2). For example, if a patient exhibits a hard end feel with elbow extension and resistance before pain, aggressive stretching and joint mobilization techniques can be initiated. Conversely, pain exhibited before resistance and an empty or spasm end feel would be managed with more gentle stretching and attempts to diminish the pain before aggressive mobilization interventions are performed.

TABLE 8–2.
Pain-Resistance Sequence

Condition	Lesion type and management
Pain before resistance	Acute lesion, active inflammatory response; treatment focus on decreasing pain; mild stretching
Pain with resistance	Subacute lesion, mild inflammation present; treatment focus on moderate stretching
Resistance before pain	Chronic lesion, no inflammatory response present; vigorous stretching

Phase 2

Phase two, the intermediate phase, emphasizes the advancement of elbow mobility, improvement of strength and endurance, and of neuromuscular control of the elbow complex. The criteria to progress to this phase include (1) full range of motion, (2) minimal pain and tenderness, and (3) a "good" manual muscle test grade for the elbow flexors and extensors. If the patient has not passed these criteria, phase I activities would be continued until the criteria for progression are met.

In phase 2, stretching exercises are continued to maintain elbow extension and flexion, as well as pronation and supination. Elbow extension and forearm pronation are critical to the elbow, making its flexibility paramount. Wrist flexor and extensor stretching is performed, along with shoulder stretching exercises to maintain the normal flexibility of the total arm complex, thus preparing the athlete for the eventual return to sporting activities.

Strengthening exercises are advanced with use of isotonic contractions of the arm musculature. Dumbbell isotonic progressive resistive exercises are performed for the biceps, triceps, pronators and supinators, and the wrist flexor-extensor musculature. Also, a strengthening program for the complex musculature of the shoulder is used during this phase of rehabilitation. In this program, the rotator cuff musculature is emphasized, with special focus on the abductors and external rotators. The concepts of total arm strength and of proximal stability for distal mobility are stressed to ensure adequate neuromuscular performance and muscular strength and power in the performance of all upper extremity activities. To enhance these concepts, neuromuscular control exercises are performed for the elbow and shoulder muscular complexes. These exercises include proprioceptive neuromuscular facilitation exercises such as performance of diagonal patterns with rhythmic stabilization and slow reversal holds to improve control of the elbow musculature.

Phase 3

Phase 3, the advanced strengthening phase, is directed toward progressively increasing activities to prepare the patient for unrestricted functional participation. The specific goals of this phase are to increase the patient's total arm strength, power, endurance, and neuromuscular control and to prepare the patient for a gradual return to functional activities, such as strenuous work or sport training.

The criteria that must be fulfilled before entering this phase are (1) full, nonpainful range of motion, (2) no pain or tenderness; and (3) strength that is 70% of the contralateral side. Because of the explosive and aggressive movements required to perform these exercises, these criteria should be fulfilled before initiation of the specific exercises of this phase.

Advanced strengthening exercises specific for the patient's activity or position are emphasized during this phase. The exercises generally include higher demand strengthening exercises, such as high speed–high energy strengthening and eccentric muscular contractions performed in functional positions. With these strengthening exercises, neuromuscular control and coordination drills are initiated to facilitate the functional return of the patient to symptom-free functional activities. Thus, plyometrics or stretch shortening exercises are performed for the shoulder and arm musculature to enhance muscular performance.[33]

For the elbow of a thrower, a large emphasis is placed on the biceps musculature. The biceps muscle is an important stabilizer during the follow-through phase of throwing, when the elbow flexors must eccentrically contract to decelerate the elbow and prevent hyperextension or the potentially pathologic abutting of the olecranon into its fossa.[2, 8] The elbow flexors are exercised by using elastic exercise tubing to emphasize slow and fast muscular contractions in both a concentric and especially an eccentric fashion (Fig 8–4). Plyometrics are also performed for the biceps by using exercise tubing.[32] This exercise is initiated with the elbow flexed entirely and the shoulder flexed to about 60° with the exercise tubing in hand. The athlete then releases this isometric hold, allowing

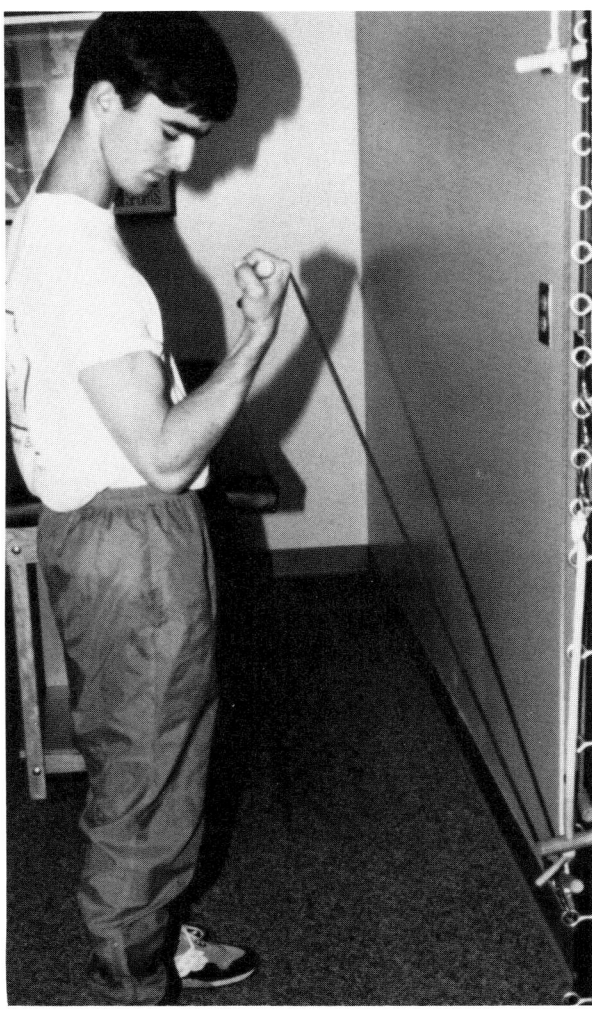

FIG 8–4. Elbow flexion performed with exercise tubing provides concentric and eccentric muscle contraction.

the elbow to extend rapidly (eccentric phase); as elbow extension is reached, the movement is quickly reversed back into elbow flexion to complete the plyometric activity (concentric phase). The basic concept of plyometrics is to use the eccentric phase (the loading phase) to cause a stretch on the muscle spindle. This stretch affords the muscle the ability to perform a facilitated concentric contraction.

Triceps exercises are performed to simulate their role during the acceleration phase of throwing.[13] The triceps are exercised concentrically by using exercise tubing activities for both slow and fast contractions. Also, the wrist flexor-pronator muscle group is aggressively exercised because of its importance in medial stabilization of the elbow during throwing. This is performed by using a concentric-eccentric muscle contraction with exercise tubing. The elbow extensors and supinators must also be exercised. All exercise tubing activities are performed for three to four sets of 10 to 15 repetitions each, alternating sets of slow and fast speeds.

An aggressive exercise program for the rotator cuff musculature and the shoulder complex musculature is also used. To accomplish the goal of total arm strength, the throwing athlete is required to follow the "thrower's 10"[31] exercise program for shoulder girdle musculature.[33] These exercises, intended to exercise the muscle groups of the glenohumeral, scapulothoracic, and elbow complex joints, include the following:
- Dumbbell exercises for the deltoid and supraspinatus musculature
- Prone horizontal shoulder abduction
- Prone shoulder extension
- Internal rotation at 90° abduction of the shoulder, with tubing
- External rotation at 90° abduction of the shoulder, with tubing
- Elbow flexion-extension exercises (exercise tubing)
- Serratus anterior strengthening and progressive pushups
- Diagonal D_2 pattern for shoulder extension with exercise tubing
- Diagonal pattern D_2 flexion with tubing
- Dumbbell wrist extension-flexion

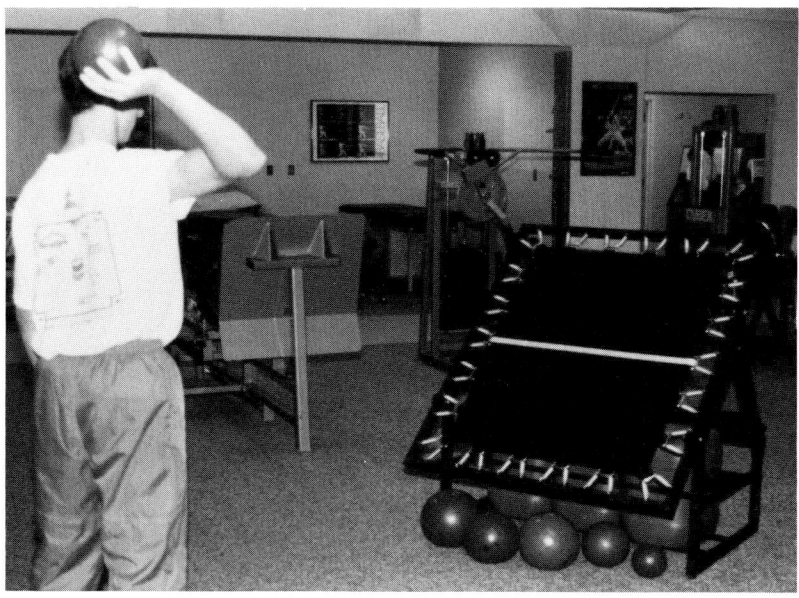

FIG 8–5. Plyometric training with a Plyoball and Plyoback, to simulate throwing motion. This drill is called a one-hand overhead baseball throw.

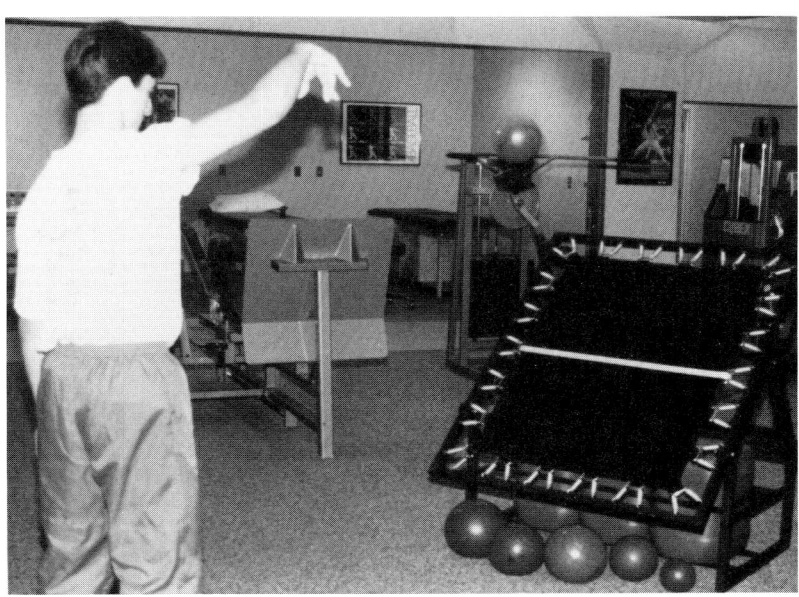

FIG 8-6. Plyometric exercise: a 2-lb Plyoball is thrown into the Plyoback with a baseball throwing motion.

Also in this phase, advanced exercises with a weighted medicine ball (Plyoball*) can be initiated. These are total body exercises that train the athlete to transfer energy and stabilize the affected area; they also teach acceleration-deceleration concepts for the throwing arm. In these exercises, a Plyoball and Plyoback exercise equipment (Functionally Integrated Technology, Dublan, Calif.). The athlete throws a 2-lb Plyoball ball against the screen; after the ball bounces back, the patient catches it one-handed and quickly throws the ball back into the Plyoback screen. The movement is performed as rapidly as possible, and the ball should be in the athlete's hand for only a minimal time (Fig 8-5). Plyoball exercises also include the wall throw (Fig 8-6), soccer throw (Fig 8-7), chest pass (Fig 8-8), and side-to-side throw (Fig 8-9), to name a few. A complete description of a wide variety of upper extremity plyometric activities can be found in an article by Wilk et al.[32]

Phase 4

The last phase of rehabilitation for the throwing elbow is the return to activity phase. The goal is to assure that adequate motion, strength, and functional capabilities have been achieved. Progressive functional drills are performed to prepare the athlete to return to the specific sport or position. For a throwing athlete, an interval throwing program is used to ensure a gradual progression to unrestricted throwing activities (Tables 8-3 and 8-4). For a golfer, an interval program (Table 8-5) is used that gradually increases the number of swings and gradually increases the distance of the golf club. The interval tennis program (Tables 8-6 and 8-7) uses the concept of number of strokes and type of strokes. The principle of this inteval program is to increase progressively the demands on the shoulder, elbow, and arm by controlling the intensity, duration, and frequency of the number of swings or throws performed and the distance used.

Before an athlete is allowed to return to competitive sports, specific criteria must be met. These criteria are (1) full range of motion, (2) no pain or tenderness, (3) fulfillment of an isokinetic test with set criteria, and (4) a satisfactory clinical examination.

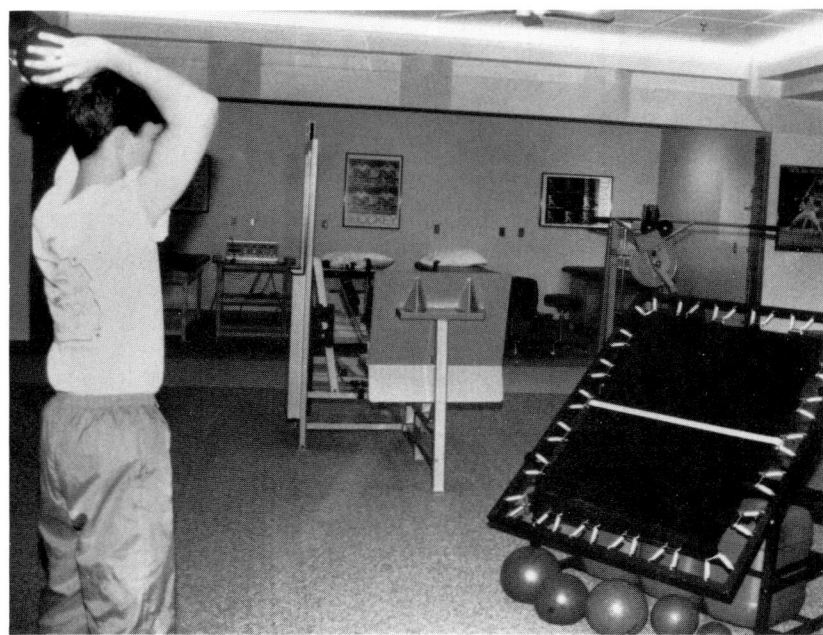

FIG 8–7. Plyometric exercise: demonstration of the soccer throw with a 2-lb Plyoball. This results in a stretch for both the shoulder and elbow musculature.

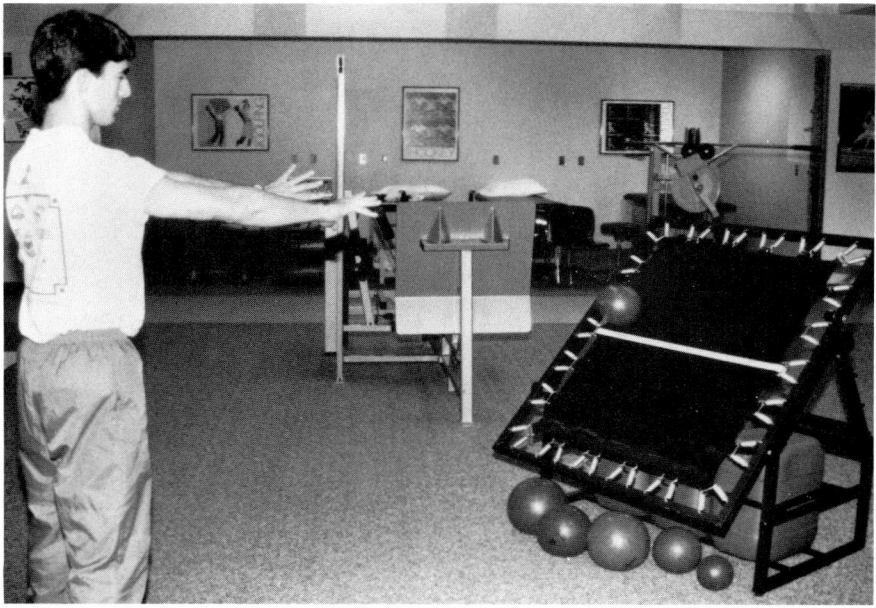

FIG 8–8. Plyometric exercise: demonstration of the two-hand chest pass.

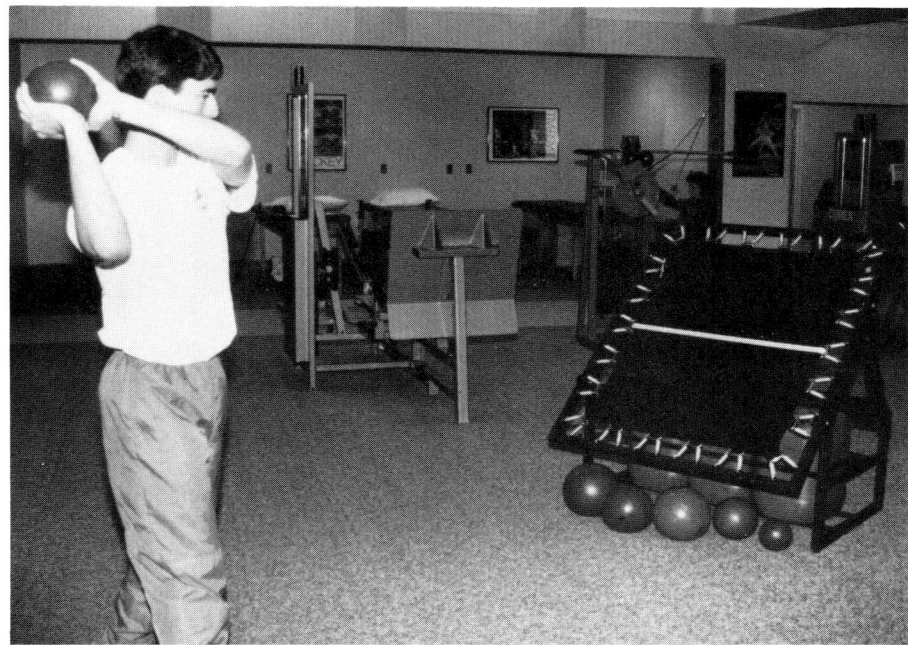

FIG 8–9. Plyometric exercise: a two-hand side-to-side pass of a 4-lb Plyoball into a Plyoback. This device is employed to enhance the transfer of kinetic energy from the legs and trunk to the arm.

TABLE 8–3.
Interval Throwing Program: Phase 1

45-foot phase	60-foot phase	90-foot phase	120-foot phase	150-foot phase
Step 1	*Step 3*	*Step 5*	*Step 7*	*Step 9*
• Warm-up throwing	• Warm-up throwing	• Warm-up throwing	• Warm-up throwing	• Warm-up throwing
• 25 throws at 45 ft	• 25 throws at 60 ft	• 25 throws at 90 ft	• 25 throws at 120 ft	• 25 throws at 150 ft
• Rest 15 minutes	• Rest 15 minutes	• Rest 15 minutes	• Rest 15 minutes	• Rest 15 minutes
• Warm-up throwing	• Warm-up throwing	• Warm-up throwing	• Warm-up throwing	• Warm-up throwing
• 25 throws at 45 ft	• 25 throws at 60 ft	• 25 throws at 90 ft	• 25 throws at 120 ft	• 25 throws at 150 ft
Step 2	*Step 4*	*Step 6*	*Step 8*	*Step 10*
• Warm-up throwing	• Warm-up throwing	• Warm-up throwing	• Warm-up throwing	• Warm-up throwing
• 25 throws at 45 ft	• 25 throws at 60 ft	• 25 throws at 90 ft	• 25 throws at 120 ft	• 25 throws at 150 ft
• Rest 10 minutes	• Rest 10 minutes	• Rest 10 minutes	• Rest 10 minutes	• Rest 10 minutes
• Warm-up throwing	• Warm-up throwing	• Warm-up throwing	• Warm-up throwing	• Warm-up throwing
• 25 throws at 45 ft	• 25 throws at 60 ft	• 25 throws at 90 ft	• 25 throws at 120 ft	• 25 throws at 150 ft
• Rest 10 minutes	• Rest 10 minutes	• Rest 10 minutes	• Rest 10 minutes	• Rest 10 minutes
• Warm-up throwing	• Warm-up throwing	• Warm-up throwing	• Warm-up throwing	• Warm-up throwing
• 25 throws at 45 ft	• 25 throws at 60 ft	• 25 throws at 90 ft	• 25 throws at 120 ft	• 25 throws at 150 ft
180-foot phase				
Step 11	*Step 12*	*Step 13*	*Step 14*	
• Warm-up throwing	• Warm-up throwing	• Warm-up throwing	• Begin throwing off the mound or return to respective position	
• 25 throws at 180 ft	• 25 throws at 180 ft	• 25 throws at 180 ft		
• Rest 15 minutes	• Rest 10 minutes	• Rest 10 minutes		
• Warm-up throwing	• Warm-up throwing	• Warm-up throwing		
• 25 throws at 180 ft	• 25 throws at 180 ft	• 25 throws at 180 ft		
	• Rest 10 minutes	• Rest 10 minutes		
	• Warm-up throwing	• Warm-up throwing		
	• 25 throws at 180 ft	• 25 throws at 180 ft		

TABLE 8–4.
Interval Throwing Program: Phase 2

Stage 1: Fastball Only
- Step 1: Interval throwing*
  15 throws off mount at 50%†
- Step 2: Interval throwing
  30 throws off mound at 50%
- Step 3: Interval throwing
  45 throws off mound at 50%
- Step 4: Interval throwing
  60 throws off mound at 50%
- Step 5: Interval throwing
  30 throws off mound at 75%
- Step 6: 30 throws off mound at 75%
  45 throws off mound at 50%
- Step 7: 45 throws off mound at 75%
  15 throws off mound at 50%
- Step 8: 60 throws off mound at 75%

Stage 2: Fastball Only
- Step 9: 45 throws off mound at 75%
  15 throws in batting practice
- Step 10: 45 throws off mound at 75%
  30 throws in batting practice
- Step 11: 45 throws off mound at 75%
  45 throws in batting practice

Stage 3
- Step 12: 30 throws off mound at 75% (warm-up)
  15 throws off mound at 50% (breaking balls)
  45-60 throws in batting practice (fastball only)
- Step 13: 30 throws off mound at 75%
  30 breaking balls at 75%
  30 throws in batting practice
- Step 14: 30 throws off mound at 75%
  60-90 throws in batting practice at 25% (breaking balls)
- Step 15: Simulated game progressing by 15 throws per workout.

*Use interval throwing to 120 ft as warm-up.
†All throwing off the mound should be done in the presence of a pitching coach to stress proper mechanics. A speed gun should be used to control effort.

TABLE 8–5.
Interval Golf Program*

Week	Monday	Wednesday	Friday
1	10 putts 10 chips 5-min rest 15 chips	15 putts 15 chips 5-min rest 25 chips	20 putts 20 chips 5-min rest 20 putts 20 chips 5-min rest 10 chips 10 short irons
2	20 chips 10 short irons 5-min rest 10 short irons	20 chips 15 short irons 10-min rest 15 short irons 15 chips putting	15 short irons 10 medium irons 10-min rest 20 short irons 15 chips
3	15 short irons 15 medium irons 10-min rest 5 long irons 15 short irons 15 medium irons 10-min rest 20 chips	15 short irons 10 medium irons 10 long irons 10-min rest 10 short irons 10 medium irons 5 long irons 5 wood	15 short irons 10 medium irons 10 long irons 10-min rest 10 short irons 10 medium irons 10 long irons 10 wood
4	15 short irons 10 medium irons 10 long irons 10 drives 15-min rest Repeat	9 holes	9 holes
5	9 holes	9 holes	18 holes

*Perform flexing exercises before hitting, and use ice after play. Chips should be performed with a pitching wedge. Short irons, W, 9, 8; medium irons, 7, 6, 5; long irons, 4, 3, 2; woods, 3, 5; drives should be performed with a driver.

TABLE 8-6.
Interval Tennis Program*

Week	Monday	Wednesday	Friday
1	12 FH	15 FH	15 FH
	8 BH	8 BH	10 BH
	10-min rest	10-min rest	10-min rest
	13 FH	15 FH	15 FH
	7 BH	7 BH	10 BH
2	25 GH	30 FH	30 FH
	15 BH	20 BH	25 BH
	10-min rest	10-min rest	10-min rest
	25 FH	30 RH	30 FH
	15 BH	20 BH	10 OH
3	30 FH	30 FH	30 FH
	25 BH	25 BH	30 BH
	10 OH	15 OH	15 OH
	10-min rest	10-min rest	10-min rest
	30 FH	30 FH	30 FH
	25 BH	25 BH	15 OH
	10 OH	15 OH	10-min rest
			30 FH
			30 BH
			15 OH
4	30 FH	30 FH	30 FH
	30 BH	30 BH	30 BH
	10 OH	10 OH	10 OH
	10-min rest	10-min rest	10-min rest
	Play 3 games	Play set	Play 1½ sets
	10 FH	10 FH	10 FH
	10 BH	10 BH	10 BH
	5 OH	5 OH	3 OH

*BH, backhand grand strokes; RH, forehand grand strokes; OH, overhead shots.

TABLE 8-7.
Interval Tennis Program*

Day of Week	Week 1	Week 2	Week 3	Week 4
Monday	12 FH	25 FH	30 FH	30 FH
	8 BH	15 BH	25 BH	30 BH
	10-min rest	10-min rest	10 OH	10 OH
	13 FH	25 FH	10-min rest	10-min rest
	7 BH	15 BH	30 FH	Play 3 games
			25 BH	10 FH
			10 OH	10 BH
				5 OH
Wednesday	15 FH	30 FH	30 FH	30 FH
	8 BH	20 BH	25 BH	30 BH
	10-min rest	10-min rest	15 OH	10 OH
	15 FH	30 FH	10-min rest	10-min rest
	7 BH	20 BH	30 FH	Play set
			25 BH	10 FH
			15 OH	10 BH
				5 OH
Friday	15 FH	30 FH	30 FH	30 FH
	10 BH	25 BH	30 BH	30 BH
	10-min rest	10-min rest	15 OH	10 OH
	15 FH	30 FH	10-min rest	10-min rest
	10 BH	15 BH	30 FH	Play 1½ sets
		10 OH	15 OH	10 FH
			10-min rest	10 BH
			30 FH	3 OH
			30 BH	
			15 OH	

*BH, backhand ground strokes; FH, forehand ground strokes; OH, overhead shots.

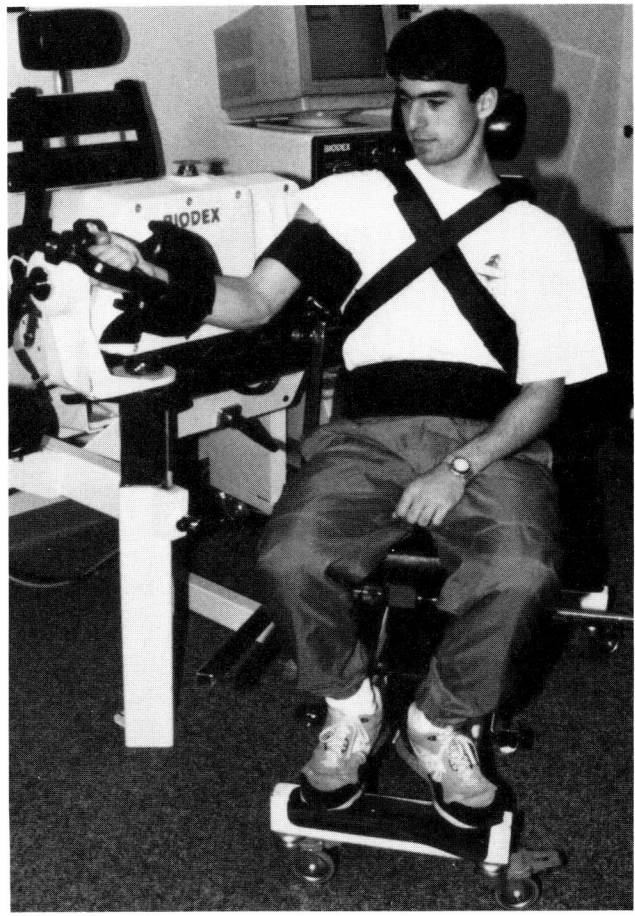

FIG 8–10. Isokinetic testing of the elbow flexors-extensors in the seated, stabilized position.

The specific criteria of the isokinetic test are part of an ongoing study we are concurrently conducting. Routinely, the throwing elbow is tested at 180°/sec and 300°/sec in the seated position (Fig 8–10). The bilateral comparison indicates the elbow flexors of the throwing arm being 10% to 20% stronger, and the dominant extensors being 5% to 15% stronger in side comparison with those in the nonthrowing arm. In addition, the flexor-extensor ratio should be 70% to 80% at 180°/sec and 63% to 69% at 300°/sec for the throwing arm. This data is useful in providing objective information regarding the muscular performance of the thrower.

REHABILITATION FOLLOWING SPECIFIC ARTHROSCOPIC PROCEDURES

Debridement

The specific rehabilitation protocols for postsurgical procedures of the elbow can be found in Tables 8–8 through 8–10. One of the common arthroscopic procedures performed in the elbow is debridement, with or without removal of osteophytes. The actual time frames for rehabilitation following this surgical procedure can be found in Table 8–8.

TABLE 8-8.
Postoperative Rehabilitative Protocol for Elbow Arthroscopy Patients

I. **Initial phase** (week 1)
   Goals: Full wrist and elbow range of motion, decreased swelling, and pain, retardation of muscle atrophy
   A. Day of surgery
      1. Begin gently moving elbow in bulky dressing
   B. Postoperative days 1–2
      1. Remove bulky dressing: replace with elastic bandages
      2. Immediate postoperative hand, wrist, and elbow exercises
         a) Putty working-grip strengthening
         b) Wrist flexor stretching
         c) Wrist extensor stretching
         d) Wrist curls
         e) Reverse wrist curls
         f) Neutral wrist curls
         g) Pronation-supination
         h) A/active assertive ROM elbow extension-flexion
   C. Postoperative days 3–7
      1. Passive ROM elbow extension flexion (motion to tolerance)
      2. Begin progressive resistive exercises with 1-lb weight
         a) Wrist curls
         b) Reverse wrist curls
         c) Neutral wrist curls
         d) Pronation-supination
         e) Broomstick roll-up

II. **Intermediate Phase** (weeks 2–4)
   Goals: Improve muscular strength and endurance and normalize joint arthrokinematics
   A. Week 2: Range of motion exercises (overpressure into extension)
      1. Addition of biceps curl and triceps extension
      2. Continue to progress progressive resistive exercises: weight and repetitions as tolerable
   B. Week 3: Full range of motion is accomplished in 10–12 days
      1. Initiate biceps and triceps eccentric exercise program
      2. Initiate rotator cuff exercise program
         a) External rotators
         b) Internal rotators
         c) Deltoid
         d) Supraspinatus
         e) Scapulothoracic strengthening

III. **Advanced Phase** (weeks 4–6)
   Goals: Preparation of athlete for return to functional activities
   Criteria to progress to advanced phase: full nonpainful range of motion, no pain or tenderness, satisfactory clinical examination
   A. Weeks 3–6
      1. Continue maintenance program, emphasizing muscular strength, endurance, and flexibility
      2. Initiate interval throwing program phase I

IV. **Return to Activity Phase** (weeks 7–12)
   Goals: Gradual return to functional activities, and further strengthening of upper extremity
   A. Week 7
      1. Initiate competitive sport activities
      2. Continue throwers 10 program
      3. Continue flexibility exercises (especially elbow extension stretches)
      4. Continue forearm supination-pronation
      5. Continue all wrist and elbow exercises

TABLE 8-9.
Elbow Rehabilitation Following Arthroscopic Chondroplasty

I. **Phase 1:** Immediate motion phase
   Goals: Improve range of motion, retard muscular atrophy, decrease pain and inflammation
   A. Day 1-3
      - Range of motion to tolerance (extension-flexion and supination-pronation)
      - Gentle overpressure into extension
      - Wrist flexion-extension stretches
      - Gripping exercises (putty)
      - Isometrics: elbow extension-flexion
      - Isometrics: wrist extension-flexion
      - Compression dressing, ice 4-5 times a day
   B. Day 4-10
      - Range of motion to tolerance (at least 10°-90°)
      - Overpressure into extension
      - Joint mobilization to reestablish range of motion
      - Wrist flexion-extension stretches
      - Continue isometrics for wrist and elbow
      - Continue use of ice and compression to control swelling
   C. Day 12-14
      - Full passive range of motion
      - Overpressure into extension (3-4 times a day)
      - Joint mobilization (if necessary)
      - Initiate light dumbbell program (progressive resistive exercises)
        Biceps and triceps, wrist flexors-extensors, supinators-pronators
      - Continue use of ice after exercise
II. **Phase 2:** Intermediate phase
   Goals: Improve strength, power, and endurance; maintain range of motion, initiate functional activities
   Criteria to enter phase II: full passive range of motion, strength of elbow extension-flexion (>4/5), minimal pain and tenderness
   A. Week 2-4
      - Continue passive resistive exercise program for elbow and wrist musculature
      - Initiate shoulder program (especially external rotators and rotator cuff)
      - Continue overpressures into extension
      - Continue joint mobilization
      - Continue ice after exercise
   B. Week 4-8
      - Continue all exercises listed above
      - Initiate *light* upper body program: bench press, shoulder press, etc.
      - Continue use of ice after activity
III. **Phase 3:** Advanced strengthening phase
   Goals: Improve strength, power, and endurance; gradual return to functional activities
   Criteria to enter phase 3: full nonpainful range of motion, strength > 75% of contralateral side, no pain or tenderness
   A. Week 8-12
      - Continue PRE program:
        Elbow extension-flexion, elbow pronation-supination, wrist extension-flexion, shoulder program for rotator cuff
      - Continue stretching into extension (as needed)
      - May initiate light tossing, light golf swing, light tennis program (check with physician)
      - Interval program (week 12)
      - Ice after participation in sport
   B. Week 12-16
      - Return to activities (sport) (determined by physician)

TABLE 8-10.
Elbow Rehabilitation Following Arthrolysis

I. **Phase 1:** Immediate motion phase
   Goals: Improve range of motion, reestablish full passive extension, retard muscular atrophy, decrease pain and inflammation
   A. Day 1-3
      - Range of motion to tolerance (elbow extension-flexion) (2 sets of 10 hourly)
      - Overpressure into extension (at least 10°)
      - Joint mobilization
      - Gripping exercises with putty
      - Isometrics for wrist and elbow
      - Compression and ice hourly
   B. Day 4-9
      - Range of motion extension-flexion (at least 5°-120°)
      - Overpressure into extension: 5-lb weight, elbow in full extension (4-5 times daily)
      - Joint mobilization
      - Continue isometrics and gripping exercises
      - Continue use of ice
   C. Day 10-14
      - Full passive range of motion
      - Range of motion exercises (2 sets of 10) hourly
      - Stretch into extension
      - Continue isometrics

II. **Phase 2:** Motion maintenance phase
    Goals: Maintain full range of motion, gradually improve strength, decrease pain and inflammation
    A. Week 2-4
       - Range of motion exercises (4-5 times daily)
       - Overpressure into extension—stretch for 2 minutes (3-4 times daily)
       - Initiate PRE program (light dumbbells): elbow extension-flexion, wrist extension-flexion
       - Continue use of ice after exercise
    B. Week 4-6
       - Continue all exercises listed above
       - Initiate interval sport program

After elbow arthroscopy, the immediate and primary goal is to reestablish full wrist and elbow range of motion as quickly and expeditiously as possible. Immediately after surgery, the emphasis is placed on full elbow extension to prevent the formation of an elbow flexion contracture. A bulky compression dressing is used to control effusion of the elbow. During the first week, isometric strengthening exercises are used to retard muscular atrophy.

At the beginning of the second postoperative week, the goal is full nonpainful range of motion with an emphasis on full elbow extension. A progressive resistance exercise program is initiated to improve arm and forearm strength. During this phase a rotator cuff strengthening program is also implemented, with an emphasis on the external rotators, supraspinatus, and abductors.

The advanced strengthening phase extends from week 3 or 4 until week 8. The goals during this phase are to improve the total arm strength, power, and endurance. Also, usually during week 3 to 6, a patient may initiate an interval sport program. If a large osteophyte is removed, the functional sport program may be delayed.

With rehabilitation after elbow arthroscopy, the intention is for motion to be regained as quickly and safely as possible. In most cases this is accomplished by 10 to 12 days after surgery. A common side effect of any elbow surgery is an elbow flexion contracture; this can be minimized by an immediate motion exercise program, with an emphasis on full elbow extension. Immediately after surgery, isometric strengthening exercises can be implemented to prevent muscular atrophy. The rehabilitation following elbow arthroscopy should be aggressive toward reestablishing range of motion and strength.

Chondroplasty

The postoperative rehabilitation program following arthroscopic chondroplasty is similar to the previously discussed protocol, with a few exceptions. In this case, the rehabilitation program is slightly less aggressive (Table 8–9). We attempt to accomplish full range of motion at approximately 12 to 14 days after surgery. Initially, the motion exercises and stretching exercises are less aggressive, in an attempt to minimize joint irritation, pain, and effusion.

During weeks 3 to 8, the patient undergoes a progressive resistance exercise program for the elbow and arm musculature. The patient may progress to more aggressive strengthening exercises 8 to 12 weeks after surgery. The patient may progress to an interval program (throwing, golf, tennis) usually at 12 to 14 weeks after a thorough clinical examination by the physician. The actual time frame to return to sport activities is dependent on size, location, and degree of the chondroplasty performed.

Arthrolysis

The rehabilitation program following arthroscopic arthrolysis of the elbow capsule is aggressive in reestablishment of elbow motion. During the first week after surgery, the patient must perform hourly range of motion exercises, with special attention paid to full elbow extension. During the second week, usually by 10 to 14 days, full passive range of motion should be accomplished, with the ultimate goal of full range of motion by 7 to 10 days after surgery. The use of the overpressure stretching exercises into elbow extension has proved extremely beneficial in accomplishment of full elbow extension. Isometric strengthening exercises are used during the first 2 weeks, with progression to isotonic dumbbell exercises during the third to fourth week. Once the patient accomplishes full range of motion, a motion maintenance program as discussed in Table 8–7 is initiated. The goal of this 4-week phase is the maintenance of full elbow range of motion, especially elbow extension. It is critical for the patient to realize that motion can be lost; therefore, stretching exercises should and must be performed for 2 to 3 months from the time of surgery. The stretching exercises should be performed for 5 minutes before and after sport activities, such as throwing, golfing, or tennis.

Arthroplasty

The rehabilitation program following arthroscopic elbow arthroplasty is similar to the arthroscopic chondroplasty protocol, with the latter being more conservative in most cases. This procedure is commonly performed for a posterior compartment osteophyte, as found with valgus extension overload syndrome. When this is the case, elbow extension often is slow to return, as outlined in Table 8–11. Usually by 10 days after surgery, range of motion should be at least 15° to 90°, and by fourteen days, 10° to 100°. In most cases, full range of motion (0° to 135°) is not accomplished until 20 to 25 days (3 weeks) after surgery. The motion is slow to progress because of osseous structure pain and inflammation.

The strengthening program is similar to the other three previously discussed programs, with isometrics being performed during the first 2 weeks and isotonic strengthening being initiated during week 3 to 4. In athletes, especially throwing athletes, a shoulder strength-

TABLE 8-11.

Postoperative Rehabilitation Following Elbow Arthroplasty (Posterior Compartment-Valgus Extension Overload)

I. **Phase 1:** Immediate motion phase
   Goals: Improve and regain full range of motion, decrease pain and inflammation, retard muscular atrophy
   A. Day 1-4
   - Range of motion to tolerance (extension-flexion and supination-pronation); full elbow extension often is not capable because of pain
   - *Gentle* overpressure into extension
   - Wrist flexion-extension
   - Gripping exercises (putty)
   - Isometrics: wrist extension-flexion
   - Isometrics: elbow extension-flexion
   - Compression dressing, ice 4-5 times daily
   B. Day 5-10
   - Range of motion exercises to tolerance (at least 20°-90°)
   - Overpressure into extension
   - Joint mobilization to reestablish range of motion
   - Wrist flexion-extension stretches
   - Continue isometrics
   - Continue use of ice and compression to control swelling
   C. Day 11-14
   - Range of motion exercises to tolerance (at least 10°-100°)
   - Overpressure into extension (3-4 times daily)
   - Continue joint mobilization techniques
   - Initiate light dumbbell program (passive resistive exercises): biceps, triceps, wrist flexors-extensors, supinators-pronators
   - Continue use of ice after exercise

II. **Phase 2:** Intermediate phase
   Goals: Improve strength, power, and endurance; increase range of motion; initiate functional activities
   A. Week 2-4
   - Full range of motion exercises (4-5 times daily)
   - Overpressure into elbow extension
   - Continue passive resistive exercise program for elbow and wrist musculature
   - Initiate shoulder program (especially external rotator, rotator cuff)
   - Continue joint mobilization
   - Continue ice after exercise
   B. Week 4-7
   - Continue all exercises listed above
   - Initiate *light* upper body program
   - Continue use of ice after activity

III. **Phase 3:** Advanced strengthening program
   Goals: Improve strength, power, and endurance; gradual return to functional activities
   Criteria to enter Phase III: full, nonpainful range of motion; strength ≥ 75% of contralateral side; no pain or tenderness
   A. Week 8-12
   - Continue passive resistive exercise program for elbow and wrist
   - Continue shoulder program
   - Continue stretching for elbow and shoulder
   - Initiate interval program and gradually return to sport activities

ening program should be initiated during week 6. In most cases, a throwing athlete can begin an interval throwing program during week 10 to 12. Again, this should be determined on an individual case basis by the physician.

INJURY PREVENTION

The prevention of injury is a key element to any sports medicine program. Prevention of elbow injuries, as with other arthrologic, pathologic conditions, begins with patient education, preventive exercises that include strengthening and stretching, and proper arm care after activity. Nirschl[19] has reported that in recreational tennis clubs, 50% of players over the age of 30 have experienced tennis elbow symptoms at some time. Epicondylitis is not limited to tennis players. It can be and is found in other sports and occupations. Lateral epicondylitis is frequently seen in tennis players, golfers, and fencers and in carpenters, plumbers, typists, and trainers. Medial epicondylitis can be frequently seen in golfers, swimmers, throwers, and manual laborers.

This overuse condition appears to characteristically affect individuals between 35 and 50 years of age. The appearance of the tendon appears to change in relationship to that of normal tendon. The abnormal tissue appears gray, shiny, edematous, and immature. Nirschl[19] has entitled this pathologic condition angiofibroblastic hyperplasia, on the basis of invasion of fibroblasts and vascular granulation-like tissue. Nirschl[19] has also classified this condition into three categories with corresponding clinical and rehabilitative suggestions.

Tendinitis of the elbow is one of the most commonly seen pathologic conditions of the elbow. In most cases it can be treated conservatively. Other pathologic conditions, such as osteophyte formation chondrodysplasia and chondromalacia may be prevented to an extent with a proper conditioning program. Athletes are encouraged to perform wrist and elbow flexion-extension and supination-pronation stretching before athletic activities. We also encourage the athlete to perform preparticipation strengthening exercises for the elbow, shoulder, and wrist musculature, including:

- Stretch wrist flexors-extensors
- Stretch elbow flexors-extensors
- Stretch shoulder musculature; anterior, posterior, inferior capsular stretches

Strengthening exercises with exercise tubing:

- Wrist extension-flexion
- Wrist pronation-supination
- Elbow flexion-extension
- Shoulder internal-external rotation
- Shoulder abduction
- Shoulder supraspinatus
- Push-ups

The athlete is encouraged to perform concentric and eccentric strenghtening movements. The eccentric muscular contraction may be beneficial in preventing the occurrence of tendinitis. These exercises can be most efficiently performed with exercise tubing. We encourage the recreational athlete (golfer, tennis player, swimmer, etc.) to perform a flexibility and strengthening program before initiation of his or her sport season and a short (10-minute) warmup before each day's participation. Perhaps through maintenance of full motion, extensibility of the musculotendinous unit, and adequate concentric-eccentric strength, some elbow conditions can be prevented from occurring.

CONCLUSION

As alluded to in this chapter, the physician, therapist, trainer, and coach must all work together as a team to achieve the common goal of returning the injured athlete to his or her sport. This chapter has outlined the basic tenets of the rehabilitation process essential to realizing this goal. Communication between all members of the team during all phases of rehabilitation is critical for appropiate ajustments in the protocols to be made for each and every patient. Though this may seem a tall task, the rewards are well worth the efforts of all of those involved in the care of injured athletes.

REFERENCES

1. Akeson WH, Amiel D, Woo SLY: Immobilization effects on synovial joints: the pathomechanics of joint contracture, Biorheology 17:95–107, 1980.
2. Andrews JR, Frank W: Valgus extension overload in the pitching elbow. In Andrews JR, Zarins B, Carson WB, editors: *Injuries to the throwing arm*, Philadelphia, 1985, W.B. Saunders.
3. Andrews JR: Personal communication, 1992.
4. Bennett JB, Tullos HS: Ligamentous and articular injuries in the athlete. In Morrey BF, editor: *The elbow and its disorders*, Philadelphia, 1985, W.B. Saunders, pp 502–522.
5. Coutts R, Rothe C, Kaita J: The role of continuous passive motion in the rehabilitation of the total knee patient, *Clin Orthop* 159:126–132, 1981.
6. Dehne E, Tory R: Treatment of joint injuries by immediate mobilization based upon the spiral adaption concept, *Clin Orthop* 77:218–232, 1971.
7. Delitto A, Rose SJ, McKower JM: Electrical stimulation versus voluntary exercise in strengthening thigh musculature after cruciate ligament surgery, *Phys Ther* 68:660–663, 1988.
8. Dillman CJ: Biomechanics of the elbow joint during throwing. Presented at the American Sports Medicine Institute, Birmingham, Ala, 1991.
9. Eriksson E, Haggmark T: Comparison of isometric muscle training and electrical stimulation supplementing isometric muscle training in the recovery after major knee ligament surgery, *Am J Sports Med* 7:169–171, 1979.
10. Gossman MR, Sahrmann SA, Rose SJ: Review of length-associated changes in muscles: experimental evidence and clinical implications, *Phys Ther* 62:1799–1807, 1982.
11. Green DP, McCoy H: Turnbuckle orthotic correction of elbow-flexion contractures, *J Bone Joint Surg [Am]* 61:1092, 1979.
12. Haggmark T, Eriksson E: Cylinder or mobile cast brace after knee ligament surgery: a clinical analysis and morphologic and enzymatic studies of changes of the quadriceps muscle, *Am J Sports Med* 7:48–56, 1979.
13. Jobe FW, Moynes DR, Tibone JE, Perry J: An EMG analysis of the shoulder in pitching: a second report, *Am J Sports Med* 12:218–220, 1984.
14. Kalteborn FM: Mobilization of the extremity joints: examination and basic treatment techniques. Oslo, Norway, Olaf Norlis Bokhard, 1980, pp 86-91.
15. Kottke FJ, Pauley DL, Ptak RA: The rationale for prolonged stretching for correction of shortening of connective tissue, *Arch Phys Med Rehab* 47:345–352, 1966.
16. Lossing I, Grimby G, Johnsson T: Effects of electrical muscle stimulation combined with voluntary contraction after knee ligament surgery, *Med Sci Sports Exercise* 20:93–98, 1988.
17. Maitland CD: *Vertebral manipulation*, London, 1977, Butterworths, pp 84–105.
18. Morrissey MC, Brewster CE, Shields CL: The effects of electrical stimulation on the quadriceps during post-operative knee immobilization, *Am J Sports Med* 13:40–44, 1985.
19. Nirschl RP: Tennis elbow, *Orthop Clin North Am* 4:787–793, 1973.
20. Nirschl RP, Morrey BF: Rehabilitation. In Morrey BF, editor: *The elbow and its disorders*, Philadelphia, 1985, W.B. Saunders, 147–152.

21. Noyes FR, Mangine RE, Barber SE: Early knee motion after open and arthroscopic anterior cruciate ligament reconstruction, *Am J Sports Med* 15:149–160, 1987.
22. Perkins G: Rest and motion, *J Bone Joint Surg [Am]* 35:521–539, 1954.
23. Salter RB, et al: The effects of continuous passive motion on healing of full thickness defects in articular cartilage, *J Bone Joint Surg [Am]* 62:1232–1251, 1980.
24. Salter RB, Hamilton HW, Wedge JH: Clinical application of basic research on continuous passive motion for disorders and injuries of synovial joints: a preliminary report of a feasibility study, *J Orthop Res* 1:325–342, 1984.
25. Sapega AA, et al: Biophysical factors in range of motion exercise, *Arch Phys Med Rehab* 57:122–126, 1976.
26. Seto JL, et al: Rehabilitation following ulnar collateral ligament reconstruction of athletes, *J Orthop Sports Phys Ther* 14:100–105, 1991.
27. Tabary JC, Tabary C, Tardiev C: Physiological and structural changes in the cat's soleus muscle due to immobilization at different lengths by plaster casts, *J Physiol* (Lond) 224:231–244, 1972.
28. Tipton CM, Mathies RD, Martin RF: Influence of age and sex on strength of bone-ligament junctions in knee joints of rats, *J Bone Joint Surg [Am]* 60:230–236, 1978.
29. Warren CG, Lehmann JF, Koblanski JN: Heat and stretch procedures: an evaluation using rat tail tendon, *Arch Phys Med Rehabil* 57:122–126, 1976.
30. Warren CG, Lehmann JF, Koblanski JN: Elongation of rat tail tendon: effect of load and temperature, *Arch Phys Med Rehabil* 52:465–474, 1971.
31. Wilk KE, Arrigo CA: Current concepts in the rehabilitation of the athletic shoulder, *J Orthop Sports Phys Ther* 18:365–378, 1993.
32. Wilk KE, Arrigo CA, Andrews JR: The rehabilitation program of the thrower's elbow, *J Orthop Sports Phys Ther* 17:305–317, 1993.
33. Wilk KE, et al: Plyometrics for the upper extremities: theory and clinical application, *J Orthop Sports Phys Ther* 17:225–239, 1993.
34. Williams PE, Goddspink G: Changes in sacromere length and physiological properties in immobilized muscle, *J Anat* 127:459–468, 1978.
35. Ziskin MC, McDiarmid T, Michlovitz SL: Therapeutic ultrasound. In Michlovitz SL, editor: *Thermal agents in rehabilitation*, Philadelphia, 1990, FA Davis, pp 144–155.

Chapter 9

Clinical Experience

Laura A. Timmerman, M.D.
James R. Andrews, M.D.

Arthroscopy of the elbow is a relatively new surgical procedure; consequently, there is little information regarding clinical experience. As the indications for elbow arthroscopy expand, reports on the results will become more prevalent.

In 1985 Andrews and Carson[1] first reported on results in 12 patients who had undergone elbow arthroscopy. They concluded that removal of loose bodies produced the best results and that outcomes after chondroplasties of the radial head and capitellum were less satisfactory.

In 1986 Andrews et al[2] reported on the results of 62 elbow arthroscopies with a mean follow-up of 1.6 years. Operative findings included loose bodies in 14 patients, osteophytes of the medial olecranon in 14, synovitis in 12, osteochondritis dissecans of the capitellum in eight, chondromalacia of the radial head in six, and fibrous adhesions in five. They found that 85% of the patients rated their elbows as good to excellent after surgery, with 89% returning to their preinjury level of performance. They again concluded that loose body removal and resection of posterior olecranon osteophytes offered the most successful results.

In 1988 Parisien[7] reported on the results of 25 cases of operative elbow arthroscopy; this included the diagnosis of loose bodies in 14 patients, synovial osteochondromatosis in five, osteochondritis dissecans in five, posttraumatic disorders in four, and coronoid fractures in two. There were 23 excellent and two good results. No postoperative complications were reported.

In 1990 Baker et al[3] reported on the long-term results of 50 patients who underwent operative arthroscopy; this included the diagnosis of synovitis in 17 patients, loose bodies in 16, olecranon osteophytes in nine, and degenerative joint disease in eight. They noted that the postsurgical outcome in patients with synovitis, loose bodies, and olecranon osteophytes was generally good, while results in patients with degenerative joint disease and loose bodies resulting from osteochondritis dissecans were variable.

In 1992 O'Driscoll and Morrey[5] reported on the results of 71 arthroscopies of the elbow in 70 patients, with an average follow-up of 34 months. The procedure was retrospectively analyzed with regard to diagnostic and therapeutic benefits. Overall, 73% of the patients benefited in some way. In the group of patients who underwent arthroscopy of the elbow for diagnostic purposes, 64% of the patients benefited. Seventy percent of the patients who underwent therapeutic procedures showed benefit from the treatment. They noted improvement rates of 75% for treatment of elbows with loose bodies, 80%

for debridement of flaps or cartilage, and 80% for arthroscopic debridement of osteochondritis dissecans. A 10% complication rate was reported, including three temporary transient radial nerve palsies, four cases of persistent portal drainage with negative cultures, and one case of 15° permanent flexion contracture.

CLINICAL EXPERIENCE IN A LARGE SERIES

Between 1980 and 1992, Dr. James R. Andrews collected information on the operative findings of 467 elbow arthroscopies. For the first 110 patients, this included the postoperative diagnosis; in 1986, the information was expanded to include operative findings, procedures performed, and any operative complications.

Data Collection

At American Sports Medicine Institute (Birmingham, Ala), for every elbow arthroscopy performed, a detailed data collection sheet is completed and the information is entered into a computer data base (Fig 9-1). This includes range of motion with the patient, anesthetized specific operative findings with regard to synovitis, condition of the ulnar collateral ligament, articular surface grading according to the method of Outerbridge,[6] any debridement performed, and operative complications. Review of this data sheet offers the surgeon a systematic approach to arthroscopy of the elbow joint.

Patient Population

The mean age of the patients was 26 years (range, 10 to 73 years). There were 437 males and 30 females. The majority of the patients (83%) were involved in sports; 45% of the total patient population was composed of baseball players. The remaining patients included those with posttraumatic injuries, rheumatoid arthritis, and degenerative joint disease.

Postoperative Diagnosis

The most common postoperative diagnosis (Table 9–1) was impinging osteophytes, which also encompasses the valgus extension overload syndrome involving the posteromedial osteophytes of the olecranon. Other common diagnoses included loose bodies, osteochondritis dissecans, arthrofibrosis, degenerative joint disease, and ulnar collateral ligament sprain or tear.

Operative Findings

Synovitis, often evident in a painful elbow, was the most common finding. This was most commonly located posteriorly. A pathologic lateral fibrotic synovial fringe of the elbow joint that impinges between the radial head and capitellum has been reported by Clarke,[4] akin to the pathologic plica seen in the knee. This lateral scarring was often seen in those with lateral epicondylitis, with corresponding chondromalacia of the radial head. Anteriorly, the synovitis and scarring can adhere to the anterior capsule and humerus, preventing full flexion, and posteriorly, the olecranon fossa can become filled with tissue-blocking extension.

Elbow arthroscopy is useful in the evaluation of the integrity of the ulnar collateral ligament (see Chapter 5). The clinical examination of valgus laxity of the elbow is difficult, especially in throwing athletes. With arthroscopy, the ulnar-trochlear joint can be directly visualized as a valgus stress is applied to the elbow, and the presence of laxity can be determined. This arthroscopic stress test, as described by Soffer and Andrews,[8] is both a sensitive and specific test for ulnar collateral ligament laxity. Tears or attenuation of the ligament can be detected, and the athlete can be treated with either rehabilitation, repair, or reconstruction.

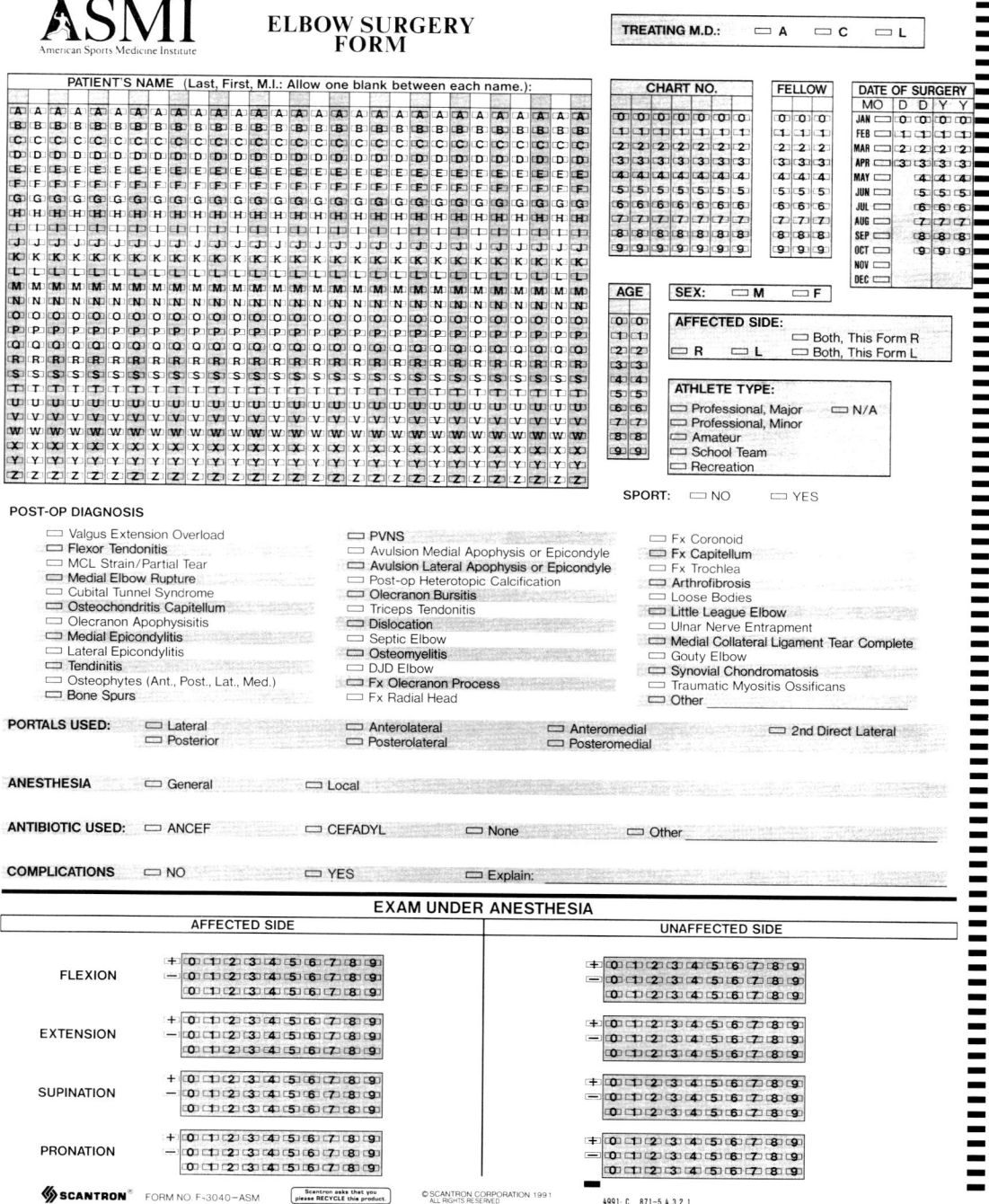

FIG 9–1. Data collection sheet used at American Sports Medicine Institute.

(Continued.)

	AFFECTED SIDE	UNAFFECTED SIDE
CARRYING ANGLE	+ 0 1 2 3 4 5 6 7 8 9 − 0 1 2 3 4 5 6 7 8 9 0 1 2 3 4 5 6 7 8 9	+ 0 1 2 3 4 5 6 7 8 9 − 0 1 2 3 4 5 6 7 8 9 0 1 2 3 4 5 6 7 8 9
VALGUS STRESS	+ 0 1 2 3 4 5 6 7 8 9 − 0 1 2 3 4 5 6 7 8 9 0 1 2 3 4 5 6 7 8 9	+ 0 1 2 3 4 5 6 7 8 9 − 0 1 2 3 4 5 6 7 8 9 0 1 2 3 4 5 6 7 8 9
FOREARM CIRCUMFERENCE	+ 0 1 2 3 4 5 6 7 8 9 − 0 1 2 3 4 5 6 7 8 9 0 1 2 3 4 5 6 7 8 9	+ 0 1 2 3 4 5 6 7 8 9 − 0 1 2 3 4 5 6 7 8 9 0 1 2 3 4 5 6 7 8 9

☐ Other Physical Exam ______

Post-op Protocol: ☐ Interval Throwing Program ☐ Elbow Program ☐ UCL Protocol

FINDINGS		PROCEDURES	
SYNOVIAL FLUID	☐ Normal ☐ Effusion/Yellow ☐ Purolent ☐ Serosang	FLUID SENT TO LAB	☐ Crystals ☐ C+ S/Gram ☐ CBC ☐ Glu/Protein
SYNOVITIS	☐ None ☐ Posterior ☐ Anterior ☐ Medial ☐ Lateral ☐ Generalized ☐ Inferior	SYNOVECTOMY/RESECTION	☐ Anterior ☐ Posterior ☐ Lateral ☐ Medial ☐ Inferior
ULNAR COLLATERAL LIGAMENT:	☐ Normal ☐ Inflamed ☐ Partial Tear-Anterior Bundle ☐ Partial Tear-Posterior Bundle ☐ Complete Tear ☐ Attenuated		☐ Observe ☐ Debride ☐ Open Repair ☐ Reconstruction Graft Type ______ Graft Size ______

ARTICULAR SURFACES: ☐ NORMAL

	RAD HEAD	CAPITEL	OLEC	TROCH	CORON		RAD HEAD	CAPITEL	OLEC	TROCH	CORONOID
Grade I	☐	☐	☐	☐	☐	Observe	☐	☐	☐	☐	☐
II	☐	☐	☐	☐	☐	Shave	☐	☐	☐	☐	☐
III	☐	☐	☐	☐	☐	Debride	☐	☐	☐	☐	☐
IV	☐	☐	☐	☐	☐	Drill	☐	☐	☐	☐	☐
Size < 1 cm	☐	☐	☐	☐	☐						
> 1 cm	☐	☐	☐	☐	☐						
Osteochondritis Dissecans		☐	☐	☐	☐	Excise ☐	Arthro Fix. ☐		Open Fix. ☐		
Anterior Osteophytes		☐	☐	☐	☐	Excise ☐					
Posterior Osteophytes		☐	☐	☐	☐	Excise ☐					

Ulnar Nerve Entrapment ☐ | Ulnar Nerve Transposition ☐

Flexor Tendonitis ☐ | Excise ☐

Loose Bodies Anterior ☐ Lateral ☐ Post ☐ Med ☐ | Removal Loose Bodies 0 1 2 3 4 5 6 7 8 9 / 0 1 2 3 4 5 6 7 8 9

Capsulectomy Anterior ☐ Posterior ☐ Medial ☐ Lateral ☐

Other Pathology ______ Other Procedure ______

FIG 9-1 (cont.).

Osteophytes were most frequently found on the posterior olecranon. These were frequently associated with a "kissing lesion" or chondral defect in the trochlea at the articulation of the posterior medial portion of the olecranon. Anteriorly, the most common location of osteophytes was the radial head, followed by the capitellum and coronoid. Abutting spurs were also seen proximal to and filling the radial and coronoid fossae of the distal anterior humerus.

Osteochondritis dissecans was most frequently located on the capitellum, followed by the trochlea and the radial head. Articular surface defects were seen on the capitellum, radial head, and trochlea, and less frequently on the ulna or coronoid (Table 9–2).

TABLE 9–1.

Elbow Arthroscopy Diagnoses in 467 Patients (1980–1992)

Postoperative Diagnosis	No. of Patients
Osteophytes	218
Loose bodies	181
Valgus extension overload	131
Medial (ulnar) collateral ligament strain or tear	70
Osteochondritis dissecans	38
Synovitis	31
Posttraumatic arthrofibrosis	30
Degenerative joint disease	18
Other	58

Operative Procedures

The most commonly performed operative procedure was excision or debridement of osteophytes, followed by removal of loose bodies (Table 9–3). Debridement of the joint surface, or chondroplasty, was performed in approximately one third of the cases. Excision of posttraumatic scarring or arthrofibrosis was performed in 19 patients. Diagnostic arthroscopy was performed in approximately 10% of the patients. Information gained from the arthroscopic examination was useful in treatment decisions. Patients often underwent an associated open procedure, including ulnar collateral ligament reconstruction or lateral extensor mass release. In patients who underwent only diagnostic arthroscopy, benefit was sometimes noted, in that the activity level and type of rehabilitation for the patient could be determined. For example, an osteochondritic lesion of the capitellum in a young gymnast could heal with a period of rest, and a partial tear of the ulnar collateral ligament without complete disruption could resolve with conservative treatment.

Complications

In this series of patients, the only complications encountered included one case of partial ulnar nerve neuropraxia, one case of olecranon bursitis, and one persistent draining posterior portal. There were no incidences of infection, vascular complications, or compartment syndrome. The ulnar nerve neuropraxia occurred during posteromedial synovectomy. The nerve was exposed and visualized arthroscopically, though none of its fibers were disrupted. The complication resolved. Early in the series, a transient median nerve block resulted after extracapsular extravasation of a local anesthetic administered in the joint after the arthroscopic procedure; this was not a full complication, but the practice was discontinued.

TABLE 9–2.

Operative Findings in 275 Patients

Synovitis		*Osteochondritis dissecans*		*Ulnar collateral ligament findings*	
Anterior	53	Radial Head	3	Inflamed	6
Lateral	8	Capitellum	16	Partial Tear	11
Posterior	184	Olecranon	2	Complete Tear	11
Articular surface defects		Trochlea	4	Attenuated	9
Radial Head	33	*Osteophytes*			
Capitellum	35	Radial Head	14		
Olecranon	16	Capitellum	9		
Trochlea	31	Olecranon	170		
Coronoid	10				

TABLE 9–3.

Operative Procedures

Procedure	No. of Patients
Excision or debridement of an osteophyte	225
Removal of loose bodies	186
Synovectomy	97
Debridement of joint surface	70
Chondroplasty	40
Debridement of scar tissue	42
Diagnostic arthroscopy	46

Outcome Studies

As noted earlier in this chapter, 467 elbow arthroscopies were performed by the senior author between 1980 and 1992. Outcome studies of several subgroups of this total have been performed.

The first clinical evaluation was a study performed and reported by Andrews et al in 1986,[2] which included 62 operative elbow arthroscopies. Most of the patients were involved in athletics. Their activities included professional and college baseball pitching ($n = 22$), football ($n = 8$), Little League baseball ($n = 5$), weight lifting ($n = 2$), racquetball ($n = 2$), golf ($n = 2$), cheerleading ($n = 1$), and karate ($n = 1$). The mean follow-up of these patients was 1.6 years for 51 men and boys and 11 women and girls. Pathologic entities treated were loose bodies in 14 patients, osteophytes of the medial olecranon in 14, synovitis in 12, osteochondritis dissecans of the capitellum in eight, chondromalacia of the radial head in six, and fibrous adhesions in five. Three patients had negative findings.

The results were rated as excellent, good, fair, or poor for both objective and subjective criteria. Preoperative and postoperative objective categories included tenderness, effusion, flexion contracture, and degree of pronation and supination. Subjective categories included pain, locking or catching, return to previous activity, and swelling (Table 9–4). A point system was used to evaluate subjective and objective categories. The patients were then given overall results ratings on the basis of accumulation of points. The cumulative objective and subjective results are summarized in Table 9–5. According to the combined subjective and objective criteria, 85% of the patients rated their elbows as excellent or good after surgery, and 89% of them returned to their preinjury levels of performance. Evaluation of the procedures performed revealed that loose body removal and resection of olecranon osteophytes produced the highest percentage of excellent and good results, followed by synovectomy, chondroplasty of the capitellum, and chondroplasty of the radial head.

Review of our clinical experience with elbow arthroscopy reveals that this certainly has been a rewarding and worthwhile technique for both diagnostic and therapeutic purposes. Obviously, the ability to use standard arthroscopic equipment in a minimally invasive manner about the elbow has many advantages. Our clinical experience indicates that early diagnosis of common elbow disorders and early arthroscopic intervention obviously gives the best results. Loose body removal continues to be the most prevalent indication for elbow arthroscopy and also has the best overall result.

In our clinical experience, the ability to remove offending osteophytes both anteriorly and posteriorly has been successful. Arthroscopic visualization allows intraoperative inspection after the osteophytes have been removed, and one can readily see the resulting decompression either anteriorly or posteriorly. The range of motion also can be inspected intraoperatively and measured. The removal of posterior osteophytes between the olec-

TABLE 9-4.
Objective and Subjective Criteria for Elbow Arthroscopy Outcome

Result	Points	Objective Criteria	Subjective Criteria
Excellent	25	No tenderness; no effusion; less than 5° flexion contracture; normal pronation-supination	No pain; no swelling; full return to prior activity; no locking or catching
Good	20	Localized tenderness; mild effusion; 5°–15° of flexion contracture; less than 20% loss of pronation-supination	Occasional pain; occasional swelling with heavy activity; occasional disability; rare locking or catching
Fair	15	Mild diffuse tenderness; moderate effusion; 16°–45° of flexion contracture; less than 50% loss of pronation-supination	Pain with moderate activity; persistent swelling with heavy activity; less than full return to prior activity; occasional locking or catching
Poor	10	Severe diffuse tenderness; severe effusion; more than 45° flexion contracture; more than 50% loss of pronation-supination	Pain with light activity; swelling with any activity; no return to prior activity; frequent locking or catching

From Andrews JR, St Pierre RK, Carson WG: *Clin Sports Med*, 5:653–662, 1986.

ranon tip and the olecranon fossa has been one of the most successful procedures. According to outcome studies, though, these procedures must be considered palliative. There is obviously a high recurrence rate associated with long-term results of 5 years or more.

Arthroscopic intervention in elbow synovial disorders has been rewarding. The technical ability to perform a rather complete synovectomy arthroscopically has been demonstrated in a number of our clinical cases, but whether open or arthroscopic synovectomy is used, the recurrence of synovitis, particularly that associated with rheumatoid synovitis, is still a possibility.

In the outcome study by Timmerman and Andrews,[9] 19 consecutive cases of posttraumatic arthrofibrosis of the elbow secondary to a fracture or fracture-dislocation treated with arthroscopic debridement were retrospectively reviewed. All patients had pain and stiffness in their elbows, and a conservative therapy program had failed in all cases. All 19 patients were followed up after surgery for an average of 29 months (range, 12 to 51 months). Scoring systems of 100 points were used to evaluate subjective (pain, swelling, locking, and activities) and objective (range of motion) results.

The average preoperative subjective score of 59 improved to 92 after surgery ($p = .0001$), and the objective score improved from 66 to 87 ($p = .0001$). Extension improved from a mean of 29° to 11°; flexion improved from an average of 123° to 134°.

TABLE 9-5.
Objective and Subjective Results

Result	Points	Objective		Subjective	
		Preoperative	Postoperative	Preoperative	Postoperative
Excellent	90–100	0	14	0	12
Good	70–89	24	39	18	36
Fair	50–69	26	7	31	9
Poor	1–49	12	2	13	5
Percentage of satisfactory results	excellent + good	39	85	29	77

From Andrews JR, St Pierre RK, Carson WG: *Clin Sports Med*, 5:653–662, 1986.

There was one failure, in a patient with severe arthritis that required subsequent arthrotomy. One patient required a second arthroscopic debridement; there were no other complications. Fourteen patients had limitations in their sports activity before surgery, and 11 were able to return to their preinjury level of activity.

This study demonstrated good to excellent overall long-term results in 84% of the patients treated with arthroscopic debridement for posttraumatic elbow arthrofibrosis. Although complete return of preinjury motion was not obtained, each patient showed a significant improvement in motion and subjective symptoms.

A 30° to 45° loss of full extension of the elbow is functionally unacceptable to most patients. Range of motion can be gained by removal of intraarticular scar as well as debridement of osteophytes and removal of loose bodies in the flexion range and the extension range. One can commonly expect to be able to improve range of motion into extension to around 10° to 15° less than full extension. This certainly affords a more functional range of motion for the elbow. We are seldom able, however, to take this amount of loss of extension and correct it to a 0° loss. There is obviously a gradual loss of function of the elbow with these procedures, because of the degenerative nature of the elbow disorder.

We are currently collecting information regarding the results of elbow surgery in professional baseball players. Seventy-five players underwent surgery between 1986 and 1990. The most common diagnoses included valgus extension overload (50 patients), ulnar collateral ligament injury (19 patients), ulnar nerve neuritis (eight patients), stress fracture of the ulna (two patients), and loose bodies only (two patients). The most commonly performed procedures included removal of posterior osteophyte of the olecranon (54 patients), ulnar collateral ligament reconstruction (11 patients), ulnar collateral ligament repair (three patients), ulnar nerve transfer (nine patients), and loose body removal (13 patients).

As one can see from the surgical procedures performed, we have been successful in combining an arthroscopic procedure with open procedures. The basic principles of the commonly used arthroscopically assisted techniques in the knee and shoulder are gradually being applied to the elbow. A good example of this is the evaluation for suspected ulnar collateral ligament injuries in throwers. Here, an arthroscopic approach is used to evaluate the continuity of the ligament,[8] and an open procedure can be used to reconstruct the ligament (see the section on arthroscopic stress tests in Chapter 5.)

One of the areas of concern relative to elbow arthroscopy and its clinical use is in osteochondrosis of the elbow joint. As noted, this is most frequently seen over the articular contact surface of the capitellum. Our approach is usually conservative, of course. Once fragmentation has occurred, our recommendation is to remove the loose and fragmented osteochondral portion of the lesion and to debride the base of the lesion, to promote a bleeding response for fibrous healing. We have had no real experience with replacement of these major osteochondral fragments by using pinning or screw fixation. Our early results with removal of the fragments and debridement of the base of the lesion has been rewarding; we have been able to readily regain elbow extension in these cases. Obviously, the ability of this lesion to heal is age dependent. With younger patients and quick diagnosis, complete healing of the osteochondral lesion with fibrous tissue is more likely. In these young people, we have seen complete healing of the capitellar lesion and a complete return to sports such as gymnastics and even some throwing activities. If patients have reached puberty and early adolescence, however, the objective and subjective results decrease. In these cases, debridement of the fragmented capitellar region is performed to improve range of motion and to prevent further degeneration of the elbow. In these cases, impact loading activities such as gymnastics and throwing should be curtailed markedly. A long-term outcome study in these specific patients is currently being undertaken. The 5-year follow-up results are not known at this time.

SUMMARY

In this large series of patients, and in the previously reported small series of results, arthroscopy of the elbow has proved to be a useful procedure with minimal morbidity. Further studies with long-term follow-up are necessary to further delineate the effectiveness of elbow arthroscopy as a technique.

The large percentage of excellent and good results in patients who have undergone correction of mechanical disorders of the elbow has been encouraging. Removal of loose bodies and impinging olecranon osteophytes offers the best functional results. Chondroplasties of the radial head and capitellum produce less satisfactory results than do the correction of mechanical disorders.

In conclusion, arthroscopy of the elbow is an effective diagnostic procedure and is effective in treating certain intraarticular problems with minimal morbidity, with rapid return to function. Attention to details is essential to prevent compromise of the surrounding neurovascular structures or damage to the delicate articular cartilage.

REFERENCES

1. Andrews JR, Carson WG: Arthroscopy of the elbow, *Arthroscopy* 1:97–107, 1985.
2. Andrews JR, St Pierre RK, Carson WG: Arthroscopy of the elbow, *Clin Sports Med* 5:653–662, 1986.
3. Baker CL, Peterson WW, DaSilva R: Operative arthroscopy: long-term follow-up. Paper presented at the 1991 American Orthopaedic Society of Sports Medicine Specialty Day Meeting, Anaheim, Calif, 1991.
4. Clarke RP: Symptomatic, lateral synovial fringe (plica) of the elbow joint, *Arthroscopy* 4:112–116, 1988.
5. O'Driscoll SW, Morrey BF: Arthroscopy of the elbow, *J Bone Joint Surg* 74:84–94, 1992.
6. Outerbridge RE: The etiology of chondromalacia patellae, *J Bone Joint Surg* 43B:752–757, 1961.
7. Parisien JS: Arthroscopic surgery of the elbow, *Bull Hosp Jt Dis Orthop Inst* 48:149–158, 1988.
8. Soffer SR, Andrews JR: The ulnar collateral ligament arthroscopic stress test, in press.
9. Timmerman LA, Andrews JR: Arthroscopic treatment of posttraumatic elbow pain and stiffness, Manuscript submitted for publication, 1993.

Index

A

Abrasion arthroplasty, arthroscopic
   for degenerative joint disease, 66, 68-70, 71-73
   for valgus extension overload, 70, 73-74, 75-77
Accessory lateral portal for diagnostic arthroscopy using Andrews' surgical technique, 49
Adhesions, elbow arthroscopy for, 8
Anatomy of elbow, 11-31
   arthroscopic, 28-31
   gross, 11-25
      anterior aspect of, 11, 12, 15
      bony, 11-12, 14-15
         intraarticular, 16-19
      neurovascular pattern of, 20-25
      posterior aspect, 11, 13-14
   portal, 20, 21, 26-28
Andrews' surgical technique for diagnostic arthroscopy, 34-53
   using anterolateral portal, 38-43
   using anteromedial portal, 43-47
   using direct straight lateral portal, 47-49
   using lateral accessory portal, 49
   using posterolateral portal, 49-53
   using straight posterior portal, 52, 53
Anterolateral portal, 21, 26, 29
   for diagnostic arthroscopy using Andrews' surgical technique, 38-43
Anteromedial portal, 20, 26-27, 29
   for diagnostic arthroscopy using Andrews' surgical technique, 43-47
   establishment of, "Wissinger rod" technique for, 61
Artery
   brachial, 22, 23, 25
   radial, 22, 25
   ulnar, 22, 25
Arthritis
   posttraumatic, elbow arthroscopy for, 7
   rheumatoid, arthroscopic synovial biopsy and synovectomy for, 87-88, 89-91, 92
   septic, surgical arthroscopy for, 8, 97-98
Arthrolysis, arthroscopic
   for elbow contractures, 74, 78-83
      case history on, 80-83
      technique of, 78-80
   rehabilitation following, 125, 126
Arthroplasty, arthroscopic
   abrasion
      for degenerative joint disease, 66, 68-70, 71-73
      for valgus extension overload, 70, 73-74, 75-77
   rehabilitation following, 126-128
Arthroscopic stress test in ulnar collateral ligament evaluation, 84-86

B

Biopsy, synovial, in rheumatoid arthritis, 87-88, 89-91, 92
Bony anatomy of elbow, 11-12, 14-15
Brachial artery, 22, 23, 25

C

Chondroplasty, arthroscopic
   for osteochondritis dissecans, 62, 65-66, 67-68
   rehabilitation following, 124, 126
Clinical experience, 131-139
   complications in, 135
   data collection on, 132, 133-134
   operative findings in, 132-134, 135
   operative procedures in, 135, 136
   outcome studies in, 136-139
   patient population in, 132
   postoperative diagnosis in, 132, 135
Complications, 101-107
   in clinical experience, 135
   initial arthroscopic portal and, 104-105
   neurovascular, 101-104
   prevention of, 105-107

Contractures
  arthroscopic arthrolysis for, 74, 78-83 (see also Arthrolysis for elbow contractures, arthroscopic)
  elbow arthroscopy for, 8
Contraindications, 9
Coronoid fossa, 16

D

Debridement, arthroscopic, rehabilitation following, 122-123, 125-126
Degenerative joint disease, arthroscopic abrasion arthroplasty for, 66, 68-70, 71-73
Diagnostic arthroscopy, 33-56
  Andrews' surgical technique for, 34-53
    using anterolateral portal, 38-43
    using anteromedial portal, 43-47
    using direct straight lateral portal, 47-49
    using lateral accessory portal, 49
    using posterolateral portal, 49-53
    using straight posterior portal, 52, 53
  anesthesia for, 34
  instrumentation for, 33-34
  Poehling surgical technique for, 53-55
  postoperative routine for, 56
Direct lateral portal, 27, 30
  for diagnostic arthroscopy using Andrews' surgical technique, 47-49

E

Evolution of elbow arthroscopy, 1-2

F

Fracture, surgical arthroscopy for, 8, 98-100

H

History, 1-2

I

Indications, 5-9
Inflammation, reduction of, in rehabilitation, 112
Injury
  acute, elbow arthroscopy for, 8
  prevention of, rehabilitation and, 128-129
Instrumentation for diagnostic arthroscopy, 33-34

J

Joint(s)
  degenerative disease of, arthroscopic abrasion arthroplasty for, 66, 68-70, 71-73
  mobilization of, in rehabilitation, 110-112

L

Lateral antebrachial cutaneous nerve, 20, 21
Lateral collateral ligament complex, 18, 19
Loose bodies, surgical arthroscopy for, 5-6, 59-63
  case study on, 61, 62-64
  technique of, 60-61

M

Medial antebrachial cutaneous nerve, 20
Medial brachial cutaneous nerve, 20, 21
Medial collateral complex, 18, 19
Median nerve, 20, 22, 23
  damage to, complicating arthroscopy, 103
Muscle(s) of elbow, 11, 12, 13
  atrophy of, retardation of, in rehabilitation, 112-113
Musculocutaneous nerve, 20

N

Neurovascular complications, 101-104
Neurovascular pattern, 20-25

O

Olecranon fossa, 16, 17
Olecranon process, 16, 18
Osteoarthritis, elbow arthroscopy for, 7
Osteochondritis dissecans
  chondroplasty for, surgical arthroscopy for, 62, 65-66, 67-68
  elbow arthroscopy for, 6
Osteochondromatosis, synovial, surgical arthroscopy for, 88, 91-93, 94-96

P

Painful elbow, undiagnosed, elbow arthroscopy for, 9
Pain reduction in rehabilitation, 112
Panner's disease, elbow arthroscopy for, 6
Pigmented villonodular synovitis, surgical arthroscopy for, 93, 96
Plyometrics in rehabilitation, 115-117, 118-119
Poehling surgical technique for diagnostic arthroscopy, 53-55
Portal anatomy, 20, 21, 26-28
Posterior antebrachial cutaneous nerve, 20, 21
Posterolateral portal, 21, 28, 31
  for diagnostic arthroscopy using Andrews' surgical technique, 49-53

R

Radial artery, 22, 25
Radial fossa, 16
Radial nerve, 24

damage to, complicating arthroscopy, 103
Radiohumeral articulation, 18
Rehabilitation, 109-129
   following arthroscopic arthrolysis, 125, 126
   following arthroscopic arthroplasty, 126-128
   following arthroscopic chondroplasty, 124, 126
   following arthroscopic debridement, 122-123, 125-126
   injury prevention and, 128-129
   phase 1 of, 110-113
   phase 2 of, 114
   phase 3 of, 114-117, 118-119
   phase 4 of, 117, 119-122
   principles of, 109-110
Rheumatoid arthritis, arthroscopic synovial biopsy and synovectomy for, 87-88, 89-91, 92

S

Septic arthritis, surgical arthroscopy for, 8, 97-98
Straight posterior portal, 28, 31
   for diagnostic arthroscopy using Andrews' surgical technique, 52, 53
Strengthening exercises in rehabilitation, 114-115
Stretching exercises in rehabilitation, 114
Surgical arthroscopy, 59-100
   for abrasion arthroplasty, 66, 68-74
      for degenerative joint disease, 66, 68-70, 71-73
   in arthrolysis for elbow contractures, 74, 78-83
   for chondroplasty for osteochondritis dissecans, 62, 65-66, 67-68
   for fractures, 98-100
   for loose body removal, 59-61, 62-64
      case history on, 61, 62-64
      technique of, 60-61
   for pigmented villinodular synovitis, 93, 96
   rehabilitation following, 109-129 (*see also* Rehabilitation)
   for rheumatoid arthritis, 87-88, 89-91, 92
   for septic arthritis, 97-98

   for synovial osteochondromatosis, 88, 91-93, 94-96
   for synovial plicae excision, 96-97
   in tumor treatment, 88, 91-96
   in ulnar collateral ligament evaluation, 84-86
Synovectomy, arthroscopic, in rheumatoid arthritis, 87-88, 89-91, 92
Synovial biopsy in rheumatoid arthritis, 87-88, 89-91, 92
Synovial osteochondromatosis, surgical arthroscopy for, 88, 91-93, 94-96
Synovial plicae excision, arthroscopic, 96-97
Synovitis
   chronic, elbow arthroscopy for, 6-7
   pigmented villonodular, surgical arthroscopy for, 93, 96

T

Trochlear notch, 16, 17
Tumor treatment, surgical arthroscopy in, 88, 91-96

U

Ulna, proximal, 16, 17
Ulnar artery, 22, 25
Ulnar collateral ligament, evaluation of, arthroscopic stress test in, 84-86
Ulnar nerve, 24-25
   damage to, complicating arthroscopy, 103
Ulnohumeral articulation, 18

V

Valgus extension overload
   arthroscopic abrasion arthroplasty for, 70, 73-74, 75-77
   elbow arthroscopy for, 7-8
Villonodular synovitis, pigmented, surgical arthroscopy for, 93, 96

W

"Wissinger rod" technique for anteromedial portal establishment, 61